The Joyous Cookbook

Also by Joy McCarthy

Joyous Health

Joyous Detox

The Joyous Cookbook

100 Real Food, Nourishing Recipes for Everyday Living

JOY McCARTHY

PENGUIN

an imprint of Penguin Canada, a division of Penguin Random House Canada Limited

Canada • USA • UK • Ireland • Australia • New Zealand • India • South Africa • China

First published 2019

www.penguinrandomhouse.ca

LIBRARY AND ARCHIVES CANADA CATALOGUING IN PUBLICATION

Title: The joyous cookbook : 100 real food, nourishing recipes for everyday living / Joy McCarthy.
Other titles: One hundred real food, nourishing recipes for everyday living
Names: McCarthy, Joy (Nutritionist), author.
Identifiers: Canadiana (print) 20190044926 | Canadiana (ebook) 20190044950 | ISBN 9780735234857 (softcover) | ISBN 9780735234864 (PDF)
Subjects: LCSH: Cooking (Natural foods) | LCGFT: Cookbooks.
Classification: LCC TX741 .M33 2019 | DDC 641.5/63—dc23

Cover and interior by Jennifer Lum
Cover and interior photography by Walker Jordan
Food and prop styling by Carol Dano

Printed and bound in China

10 9 8 7 6 5 4 3 2 1

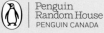

Penguin
Random House
PENGUIN CANADA

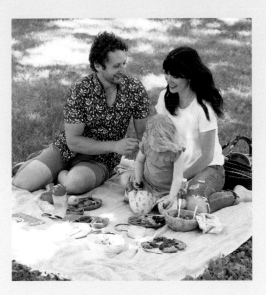

This book is dedicated to Vienna,
our daughter and little ray of sunshine
who is full of so much possibility!

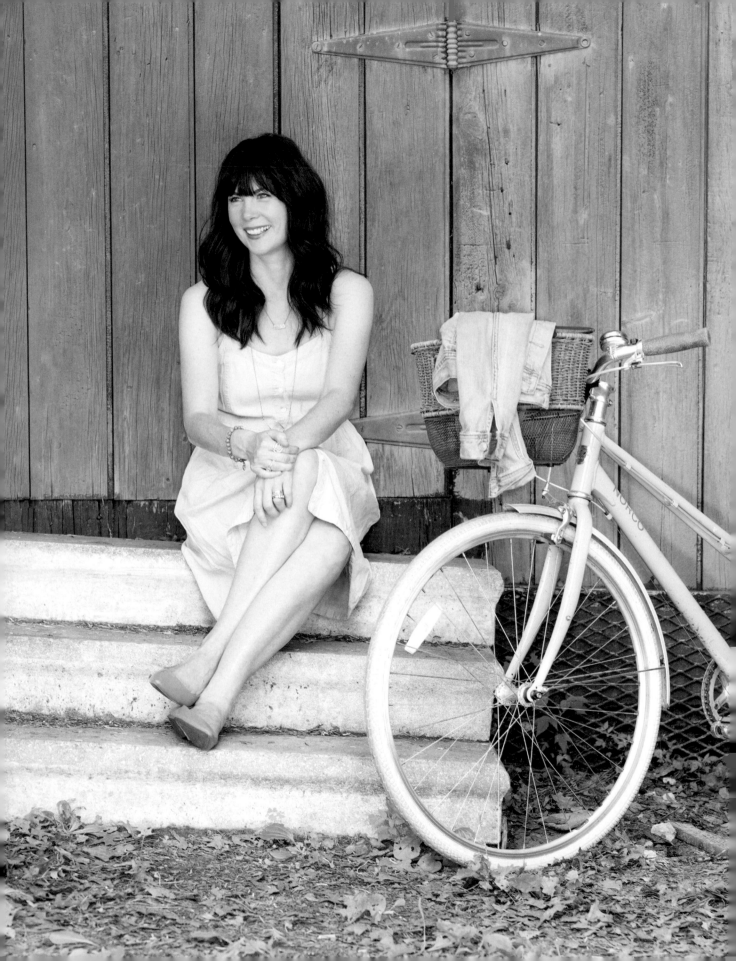

Contents

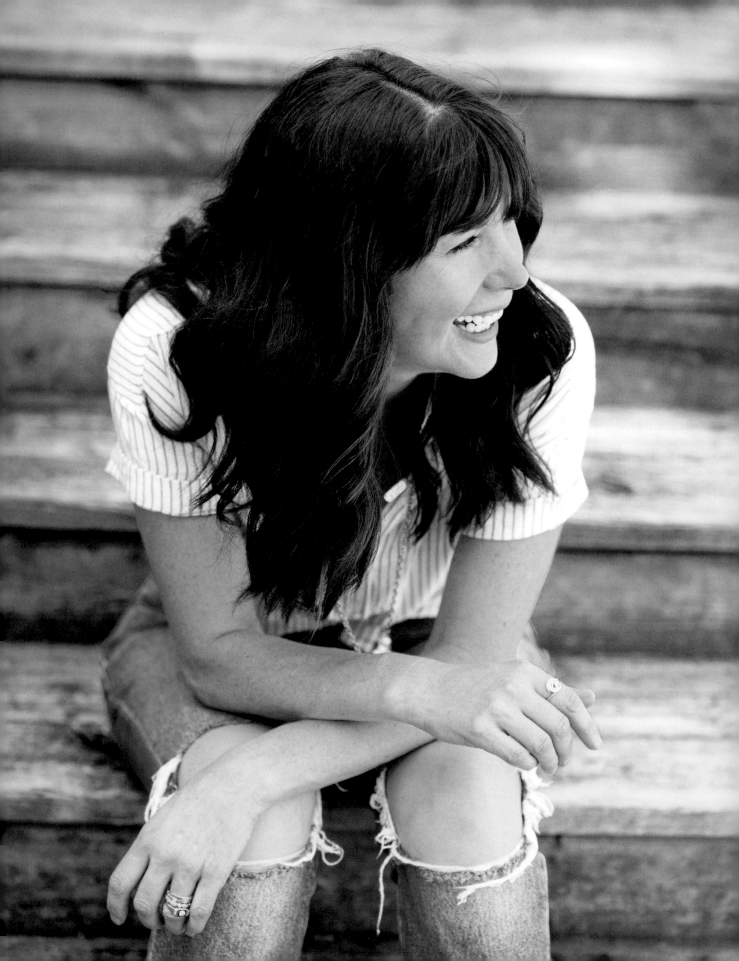

INTRODUCTION

Over a decade ago I enrolled in nutrition school to learn more about something that lit a fire in me, something that I'd been self-educating myself on for many years by attending weekend courses, reading countless books and pouring over every page of my favourite wellness magazine—that something was holistic nutrition and natural health. It was both a relief and completely terrifying to leave my career in corporate marketing with a consumer packaged food brand. Talk about a dramatic change! But somehow, I put my fear aside because I knew in my gut I was destined for this and my life would be forever changed studying what I was truly passionate about. To pay the bills, I was personal training early in the morning and into the evening, while attending school during the day. There were times that my day started at 5:15 a.m. on a freezing cold February morning jogging with a client and ended at midnight finishing my homework or cramming for a test the next day. You know what? I wouldn't change a thing!

While in school I started my blog, *Joyous Health*, excited to share everything I was learning, cooking and eating. I had healed from my own health issues (hormonal imbalance, anxiety, and digestive problems) using natural health, so I knew there must be more people out there that I could help and my blog was my communication tool. My first blog post was about a liver detox I was doing and the importance of detoxification—it was a topic that fascinated me even back then and later became my second cookbook *Joyous Detox*! The first few months I assumed no one was reading my posts. But, I continued blogging and started getting feedback from readers and it kept me going. I remember the first time a reader emailed me to tell me how much she enjoyed my blog and she was from Germany. I was floored that someone that far away found my blog and was inspired to make my chia pudding. The early days of growing my business were certainly stressful and sometimes isolating but I just keep plugging away at it because I was so grateful I was now doing what I was born to do—coach people one-on-one, teach workshops, share articles and recipes on my blog.

Fast forward to today. Life can be stressful and hectic at times, especially now that my husband, Walker, and I are parents with a very active toddler named Vienna. But we love the challenges, the highs, the lows and the in-between times of being entrepreneurs and growing our Joyous Health business together.

One thing is for sure: if I hadn't made my health a priority while in school, or the first year being a new parent, I wouldn't have had the energy to be a good mom, wife, friend or entrepreneur. Sure, there were many days I lived off smoothies and Oat, Spice and Everything Nice Balls (page 86), but something that keeps me and Walker both grounded is spending time together to share a meal at the kitchen table with Vienna. It's a priority to sit down and connect for at least one meal each day. During the week that's usually dinner, and on the weekend it's usually brunch *and* dinner.

Life gets hectic at times and we are all busy, which is why the few precious opportunities we have to slow down and connect with each other have become even more important. Mealtime is as much about nourishing our relationships as it is about nourishing our bodies.

Some of my most memorable times have been spent with family and friends over a meal. If there's one thing I've learned over my forty short years living on this planet—from my own experiences in my small but joyous kitchen, from Ma McCarthy and from such food icons as Jamie Oliver, Anthony Bourdain and Nigella Lawson—it's that food is meant to be celebrated and meals are a joyous opportunity for togetherness. I grew up in a family that valued having dinner together, and I will always make this a priority for my own family. I believe eating at least one main meal a day together is essential for a happy, nourished life. I truly hope that my recipes bring your family and friends together to share a meal.

And in my family, those meals have evolved over the years. Now more than ever in my home, food has to be as delicious as it is nutritious. A super-healthy yet bad-tasting green smoothie is just not acceptable in our home anymore. I would happily choke those back before Vienna was born, but now the three of us always share our smoothies, and there's no way a toddler is going to eat a green smoothie—or anything, for that matter—unless it tastes really good.

The recipes in this cookbook best represent what we typically eat as a family, which means they're both grown-up and kid-friendly. In other words, dishes for real living. There are plenty of gluten-free recipes and lots of dairy-free, grain-free and nut-free options. We eat things like sheep's milk yogurt and feta, so I've included these ingredients in various recipes with options if you don't eat dairy.

Even though I've designated recipes as vegan, vegetarian and so on, I don't personally subscribe to the notion that we should label ourselves based on our dietary preferences. However, if you do have dietary restrictions or allergies, you'll find it easy to identify the best recipes for you. If you feel like eating all plant-based vegan for a day or a month, then do it. If you feel like having some animal protein like salmon or chicken one day, then do it. The most important thing is that you eat foods that nourish you and help you feel your best! There's no judgment over here.

I'm so proud of this cookbook Walker and I have created for you. It was truly a joyous experience! Walker photographed (and ate) all of the recipes and continues to eat everything I make. As for Vienna, she's definitely passionate about eating too, and she's very honest. Kids either love or hate food. One thing is for sure: she loves fish, chicken fingers, pasta and pizza—all of which you'll find in this cookbook.

Happy cooking and baking, friends!

Joy
xo

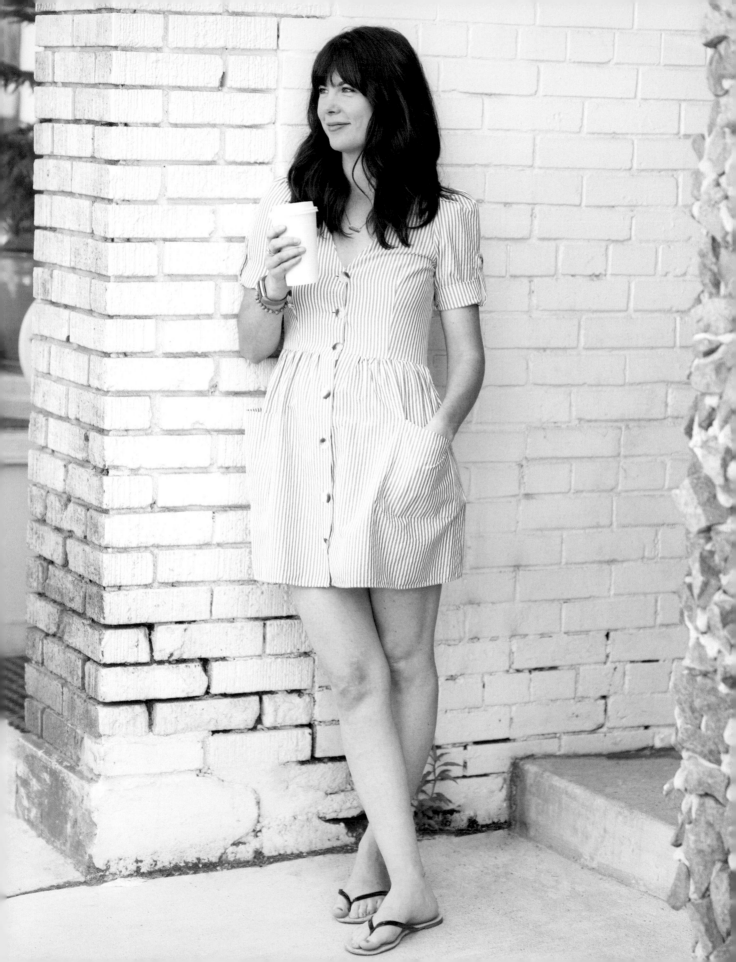

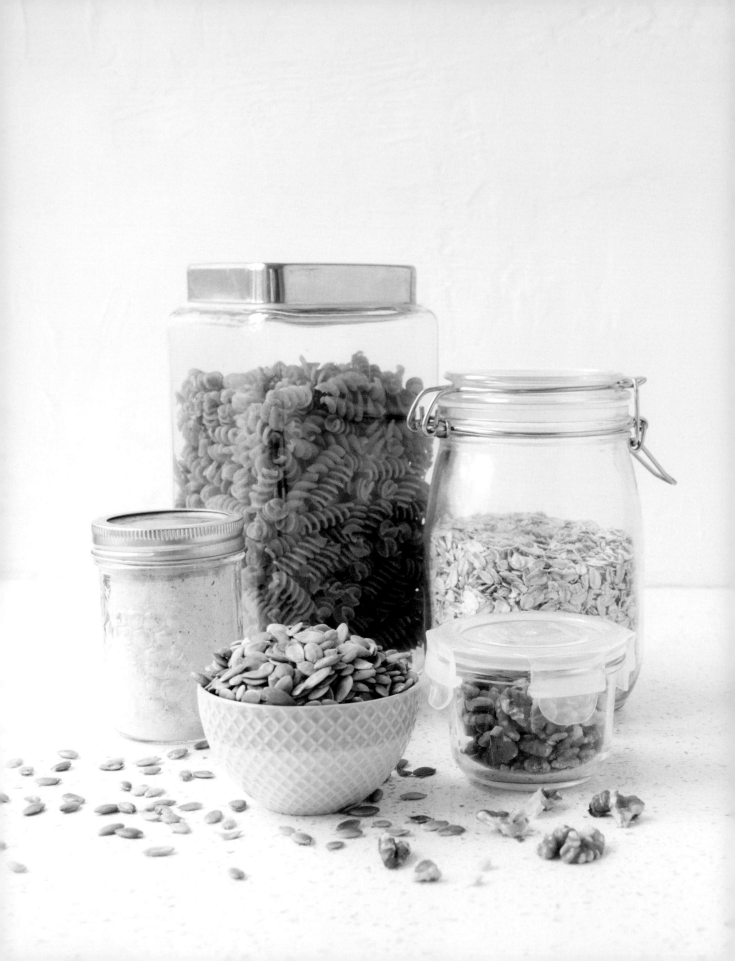

STOCKING YOUR PANTRY FOR JOYOUS MEALS

If you opened up my fridge right now, you would find lots of fresh vegetables and fruits, mostly seasonal when it's available. I do my best to buy mostly organic, and I don't typically peel a vegetable or fruit when it's organic. When you see ingredients like carrots or beets in my recipes, if you've purchased them organic then don't bother peeling unless the recipe says to or if there are a lot of bruises that you want to remove. In my fridge you would also find several jars of fermented items such as sauerkraut, pickles and of course wine! But beyond vegetables and fruits, here are the essential pantry staples that will set you up to make my recipes. Beyond the cookbook, these essentials will also set you up for years of joyous meals for a nourished life.

Healthy Fats and Oils

Good fats do more than just make food taste amazing and help you feel satiated; they also help you absorb the thousands of phytonutrients you ingest. *Phyto* means "plant," and phytonutrients are the naturally occurring medicinal compounds in plant foods that have numerous health benefits for the body. That big beautiful smoothie bowl you want to make will do a much better job nourishing you if you include some fat like avocado, coconut oil or nut milk to increase the absorption of phytonutrients in your small intestine.

Extra-Virgin Olive Oil, Avocado Oil and Toasted Sesame Oil

I use very few vegetable and seed oils such as sunflower and safflower because many of them are sold in clear plastic bottles, so they are already rancid sitting on the grocery store shelf. This is because by their very nature, being mostly polyunsaturated fatty acids, they are what we call unstable, meaning that heat, light and oxygen can be detrimental to the oil. As a general rule, steer clear of liquid oils in clear plastic bottles.

Extra-virgin olive oil is the oil I use the most. Buy the best quality you can afford, in a dark glass bottle or metal tin and preferably organic. It used to be thought that olive oil oxidized when heated, even at a medium temperature, but this is only true if you're using inexpensive, low-quality oil. High-quality oils have a much higher ratio of phytonutrient antioxidants that prevent the oil from creating dangerous free radicals. So if you're using a high-quality olive oil, you can safely cook with it.

Avocado oil can be used in place of extra-virgin olive oil, though I prefer the taste of olive oil. If you want a totally flavourless oil, then grapeseed oil is another option.

Toasted sesame oil imparts a distinct flavour to dishes, and I always keep a very small bottle of it on hand because a little goes a long way and you want to use it while it's fresh.

Coconut Oil, Coconut Butter and Coconut Milk

I purchase certified organic, unrefined coconut oil. If coconut oil doesn't taste like coconuts, it's been deodorized, which means the scent and taste have been removed, and that makes it a processed food, even if the label says it's organic. Use coconut oil in recipes where you won't mind a mild coconut flavour, like in baked goods.

Coconut butter is expensive, but it's the next best thing to dairy butter. I love to slather it on pancakes, add it to smoothies and spread it on toast. You will need to warm it a bit to make it spreadable.

I always keep BPA-free canned organic full-fat coconut milk in my kitchen cupboard for last-minute recipes, beefing up the creaminess in soups and stews without using dairy, or tossing into a smoothie for added flavour and richness.

Nut and Seed Butters

Nut and seed butters are an absolute necessity in a joyous kitchen. These healthy fats are a great way to tide you over until your next meal. That spoonful of almond butter between lunch and dinner is totally okay! Nut and seed butters can add that extra oomph to a salad dressing or they can provide just the right amount of fat to balance out the acidity of a dish. Whether you're slathering sunflower butter on toast or blending up a dip for rice-paper salad rolls, nut butters are essential. I usually have two or three different nut and seed butters in my fridge at any one time, such as tahini and almond, cashew and sunflower butters.

Natural Sweeteners

Maple Syrup

Maple syrup is my favourite liquid natural sweetener because it brings such an earthy and perfect maple flavour to dishes. Being a Canadian girl, for me it's a quintessential Canadian product! It contains minerals such as manganese and zinc, and it really shines as a source of antioxidants. But it's still a sweetener that contains natural sugar, so I use it moderately. My preference is dark maple syrup (No. 3) for a richer flavour. It's simply divine on my Stacked and Stuffed Blueberry Pancakes (page 26)!

Unpasteurized Honey

Honey is a superfood that's as ancient as they come, dating back to 5550 BC. My preference is raw and unpasteurized honey for recipes, but it must be avoided if you're pregnant and it cannot be given to children younger than two. Don't worry if the honey in your cupboard has crystallized—this isn't a sign it's gone bad. In fact, honey is a natural preservative, and provided it's pure, it will never go bad. Just warm crystallized honey over a very low heat (so you do not destroy any of its health-promoting properties) and it will become liquid again. My Honey Lemon Cayenne Elixir (page 66) is a great way to boost your immune system and soothe a sore throat.

Medjool Dates

I love adding chopped Medjool dates to a salad or using them to sweeten baked goods or provide the glue power in raw desserts—they work well to hold a nut- or oat-based cookie together. They contain 7 grams of fibre per 3½ ounces (100 g), which supports digestive wellness. Be sure not to confuse Medjool dates with the smaller honey, or Deglet Noor, dates, because a recipe like my Oat, Spice and Everything Nice Balls (page 86) will work only with Medjool dates. Dates can be the star of a recipe too, like in my Stuffed Dates Three Ways (page 85).

Coconut Palm Sugar

In recipes where I don't want to use a liquid natural sweetener, coconut palm sugar is my go-to for a granulated texture. It lends a mild caramel taste to recipes, which is perfect in cookies and pastries.

Coconut Nectar and Brown Rice Syrup

Both of these natural sweeteners are great for helping things stick together. I don't use them very often, but they are my go-to when I need sticky power. You can use either coconut nectar or brown rice syrup in my Almond Butter Rice Crispy Squares (page 220).

Baking Essentials

A kitchen that's well stocked with baking essentials makes baking much more enjoyable. I always make sure I have the staples in my pantry, like aluminum-free baking soda and baking powder, oats (both rolled and steel-cut), quinoa, dairy-free chocolate chips and various dried fruits such as Medjool dates, cranberries and raisins. Then I can whip up baked goods or a raw dessert such as my Chocolate Chip Oatmeal Tahini Cookies (page 232) without needing to go to the grocery store first.

Flours and Starches

The flours you'll most frequently find in my cookbook are buckwheat flour (and yes, despite the "wheat" it's gluten-free), almond flour (which is ground almonds and is also sold as almond meal), coconut flour and brown rice flour. I occasionally use stone-ground spelt or kamut flour. The best part about all these flours is that they haven't been stripped of their naturally occurring nutrients the way white flour and white rice flour have been.

For gluten-free baked goods, I generally use tapioca starch, also known as tapioca flour. It's made from cassava root, and it provides a crispy crust and a chewy texture. In this book I use it in the pastry for both the savoury and sweet galettes. It can also be used to thicken sauces and stews, but I typically use arrowroot starch in these instances. If you're using it to replace cornstarch, it's a 1:2 ratio—replace one part cornstarch with two parts tapioca starch.

Arrowroot starch, also known as arrowroot flour, is extracted from the arrowroot plant, and I prefer it for thickening dressings, marinades and soups. It remains stable when frozen, so your thawed leftovers won't turn goopy. Unlike cornstarch, it can be added at the very end of cooking.

For baking and raw desserts, I use organic raw cacao powder in my recipes because it's the purest form of chocolate, with the least amount of processing. It is not sweet at all—in fact it's bitter—so it's essential to combine it with something sweet. Raw cacao powder should list just one ingredient on the label: raw cacao.

Breads and Pastas

Sourdough bread is far superior to mass-produced commercial bread, which is often full of additives and other junk. My go-to bread is a crusty sourdough from my local farmers' market because it's made the way bread should be, the traditional way, with patience—letting the yeast and lactic acid work their magic. Sourdough is far more digestible because fermentation breaks down most of the phytic acid that is responsible for bloating. Less phytic acid also means the vitamins and minerals are more bioavailable, so sourdough bread is more nutritious. Its gluten is also more digestible (or you can find gluten-free sourdough). It also tends to be lower on the glycemic index. And if all that wasn't enough to persuade you, it tastes amazing! I know many people who don't digest mass-produced commercial bread well and think they are gluten intolerant but can eat sourdough bread with no problem—myself included! If you're going to have my Toast Six Ways (page 45), Walker's Breakfast Sammie (page 38) or Mushroom, Asparagus and Feta Tartines (page 122), be sure to use sourdough bread.

For pasta, I recommend using a sourdough pasta—we love the Kaslo brand. (Sourdough pasta can be hard to find in stores, but you can buy it online.) I also like chickpea pasta, quinoa pasta, brown rice pasta and sprouted whole wheat pasta. Walker and Vienna both love pasta, so it's an essential in my pantry.

Herbs and Spices

I keep a wide variety of dried herbs and spices in my cupboard, such as cinnamon, nutmeg, cloves, cardamom, garlic powder, rosemary, and Italian seasoning. I buy them in small amounts for optimal freshness and nutrition. Fresh herbs are a super-simple way to boost the flavour and nutrition in any meal. My Herby Tempeh Burgers (page 179) will make good use of your herb garden! Even if you live in a small apartment, you can have a little herb garden on your windowsill. My favourite fresh herbs to add a flavour punch to recipes are parsley, cilantro, basil, mint, rosemary and dill. I keep a few kinds of salt in my kitchen, including both fine and coarse pink Himalayan salt and Celtic salt.

Fermented Foods

Fermented foods are the best superfoods for gut health. They're easy to digest and they nourish the friendly bacteria that live in your body in the trillions. Many fermented foods are now available, but the ones I use most often are tamari (buy gluten-free if you prefer), tempeh, apple cider vinegar and sauerkraut. My all-time favourite fermented food is definitely sourdough bread. If you're soy sensitive, coconut aminos are a great substitute for tamari.

Superfoods

The superfoods I use most often are raw cacao, matcha (green tea powder), bee pollen, hemp seeds (hemp hearts) and turmeric. A few local ones I use regularly are kale, beets, garlic, carrots and mushrooms. Really, you just have to go to your local farmers' market and look for what's in season, as Mother Nature provides us with such an abundance of local superfoods.

Dairy

Goat and sheep's milk products are my preference because they are less allergenic than cow's milk and easier on my digestive system. I love halloumi and feta (both made with a mix of goat and sheep's milk), soft goat cheese, goat cheddar and sheep's milk yogurt. They add just the right amount of saltiness (in the case of cheese) and fat to a recipe to really complete the flavour profile. With any recipe in my cookbook that calls for dairy, you can use a non-dairy alternative in its place or, if the recipe won't suffer, simply omit it. For example, nutritional yeast is a great alternative to Parmesan cheese because it has a very similar taste.

Ghee is one of my favourite fats for cooking. It is essentially clarified butter cooked a little longer to bring out its rich nutty flavour. You'll see it in dozens of recipes in my cookbook. You can buy it in jars, but it's so easy (and a lot cheaper!) to make it yourself. See page 43 for three different ghee recipes. It stays fresh for months.

Protein

When I plan our meals, I always consider what protein we will have for dinner. These are the animal-based foods we eat most often: fish and seafood (salmon, arctic char, trout, sole, halibut, scallops); organic chicken, eggs, ground turkey and lamb; and occasionally organic beef. I'm not against eating red meat; we just don't eat a lot of it because we buy certified organic or grass-fed meat, which is rather expensive, and so we have it less often.

As for plant-based protein, my pantry is always stocked with various beans, chickpeas, lentils, quinoa and hemp seeds. When it comes to beans, if I'm pressed for time I use BPA-free canned, and when I have more time I use dried. Most of the recipes in my cookbook use canned simply for convenience, but anywhere you see canned you can use cooked dried beans. As well, I always have on hand a couple of bottles of plant-based protein powder—in vanilla and chocolate—for smoothies.

Frozen Staples

In my freezer I have a wide variety of foods. I always keep stocked up on protein, so when I go to my local fish market I buy more than I will need for a week and freeze most of it. Or if I'm going to the farmers' market, I might stock up on chicken and lamb. I also have plenty of frozen fruits like mango, pineapple and dark berries, and veggies like peas, green beans and corn that can be used in most recipes that call for fresh. Properly frozen, fruits and veggies can be just as nutritious as fresh. Once I've opened a bag of flour, I store it in the freezer to maintain optimal freshness.

Unless I plan on eating them within a week, I store nuts and seeds such as walnuts, cashews, pecans, sunflower seeds and pumpkin seeds in the freezer in recycled glass jars. Old nut butter jars are perfect!

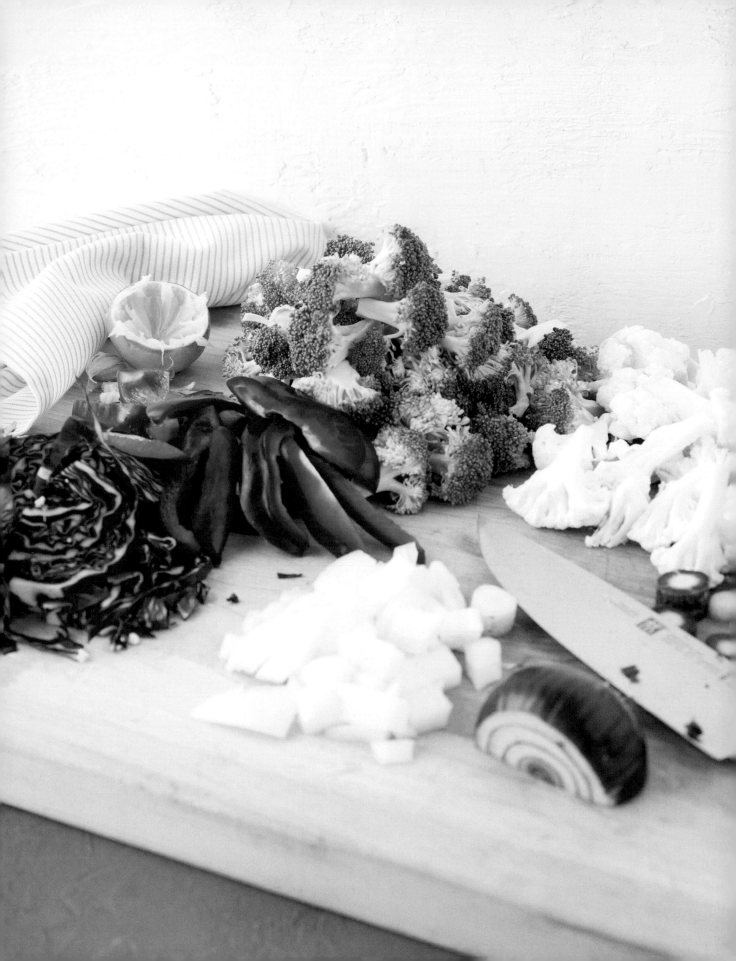

KITCHEN TOOLS AND EQUIPMENT

The equipment I list here is what I use most often and what you'll likely want to have for making most of the recipes in this cookbook. Some equipment is essential, whereas some is nice to have if you have the budget for it.

Basic Tools

Every joyous kitchen should be stocked with the following basic tools. Avoid plastic when you can for items like measuring cups and spoons. Stainless steel will last much longer.

- Measuring cups and spoons
- Vegetable peeler
- Stainless steel, glass or ceramic mixing bowls, various sizes
- Microplane grater and box grater
- Zester
- Rubber spatulas, a large one and a small one
- A couple of large wooden spoons

Good-Quality Knives

When I took culinary courses at college the most important takeaway for me was to invest in a good chef's knife (between 6 inches/15 cm and 10 inches/25 cm long). It really is an essential tool and worth the investment. You can easily spend $250 or $1,000 on a good knife, so shop around and compare prices. You don't need to spend thousands of dollars on a complete set of knives, but I do recommend that every kitchen should have at least one good chef's knife. Remember to keep it nice and sharp, so make sure you sharpen it regularly. Contrary to what you might think, a sharp knife is *less* likely to cut you. I also have a long serrated knife to get the perfect cut on crusty sourdough bread and an extremely versatile paring knife that's great for chopping up a piece of fruit I'm going to eat right away. My chef's knife is used for everything from prepping vegetables for a soup to making a big salad for dinner. (I use a paring knife for chopping up a pear to eat, but if I'm making a big salad for dinner I would use a chef's knife.)

Wooden Cutting Board

This may seem like an odd kitchen essential, but it's probably my favourite one, second only to my chef's knife. When you eat more simple, whole foods, you'll be doing more chopping, slicing and dicing. It might sound funny, but I absolutely love that crunch sound of slicing a carrot or dicing an onion. But this sound is like nails on a chalkboard—and the actual cutting is far less effective and efficient—if you're cutting on a glass, marble or ceramic cutting board. Just don't do it. Plastic cutting boards are not something I recommend unless you'd like to have plastic with your meal. They eventually break down, and when they get scratched, particles eventually come off. They may not even be visible to your eye, but they end up in your food!

Good-Quality Cookware and Bakeware

These are investment pieces that are worth every penny. I used to buy the least expensive cookware and bakeware I could find, but then I'd be replacing it every few years—not a smart investment! Now I have the same GreenPan frying pan I've been using for several years. Most of my ceramic dishes are either hand-me-downs or I've splurged on Le Creuset or Staub because I will have them for a lifetime. If you're just starting out, basics include the following:

- 13- × 9-inch (3.5 L) ceramic dish
- 8½- × 4½-inch (1.5 L) loaf pan
- Two 11- × 17-inch (28 × 43 cm) rimmed baking sheets (half-sheet pans)
- Small and large frying pans
- Roasting pan
- Regular and mini muffin tins
- Small, medium and large pots. I avoid non-stick surfaces unless they are PFOA-free.

Vegetable Spiralizer

If you want perfectly spiralized sweet potato for the Sweet Potato Veggie Pad Thai on page 108, then you'll need a spiralizer, but it's really just for looks. You could make that recipe using a vegetable peeler and making flat, wide sweet potato noodles. (Of course the cooking time may vary because a flat, wide noodle will take longer to cook than a spaghetti-like noodle.) Spiralizers are quite inexpensive, so even though I've put it in the "nice-to-have" category, they are a super-fun kitchen appliance. You just have to remember you've got it and make good use of it. My daughter loves helping me spiralize zucchini when we make my Zucchini Noodles with Turkey Meatballs (page 196).

Mandoline

For the longest time, mandolines scared me—I honestly thought I would slice off my fingers! Fortunately, they come with a safety guard to protect your fingers from the very sharp blade. Mandolines are nice to have if you want perfectly thin slices of beets to make my Rosemary Beet Chips (page 81), and they make quick work of vegetables for salads. If you buy a good-quality mandoline, you'll have it for life.

Food Processor

I use my food processor at least twice a week. If you make a lot of raw salads, raw desserts and baked goods, a food processor is definitely worth the investment because you can chop, shred, purée and make perfect Oat, Spice and Everything Nice Balls (page 86) in a snap. The food processor just makes food prep go a lot faster. Of course you can shred all the ingredients in my Shredded Brussels Sprouts Bean Salad (page 100) by hand, but a food processor will easily cut your time in half. I have a food processor that came with both a mini 2½-cup (625 mL) bowl and a large 8-cup (2 L) bowl. This is convenient, because I can make a smaller-batch recipe without getting the large bowl dirty.

High-Speed Blender

I use my high-speed blender nearly every day to make our morning smoothie. So in my kitchen, it is an essential piece of equipment. It's also handy to make pestos, puréed soups and creamy desserts like my Hazelnut Chocolate Tarts (page 228). High-speed blenders are available in a wide ranges of prices. The least expensive blenders will have a low wattage and can barely blend spinach, whereas a high-end blender can pulverize nuts with ease. A good-quality high-speed blender can last many years, making it a worthy investment, but you don't need to buy the most expensive blender on the market. A few hundred dollars will get you a decent model. Walker's cousin found an old Vitamix (the Ferrari of blenders) at a garage sale for twenty-five dollars, so if you don't have the budget for a new Vitamix, look around—you might just get lucky!

Juicer

Juicing is very seasonal for me because in the summer there is an incredible abundance of fresh fruits and vegetables at the farmers' markets. I can't say the same for the winter, when you'll never catch me sipping on a fresh juice unless I bought it from my local juice bar. It's definitely a nice-to-have small appliance, but not essential for a joyous kitchen. Also keep in mind that you can use your blender to make juice; simply strain the juice through a nut bag or a mesh strainer to remove the fibre. If you are going to invest in a juicer, I recommend a slow, or masticating, juicer because it will maintain the integrity of the enzymes in the fruit or vegetable. Centrifugal juicers, on the other hand, extract juice by forcing the fruit or vegetable through a blade, and this friction destroys enzymes.

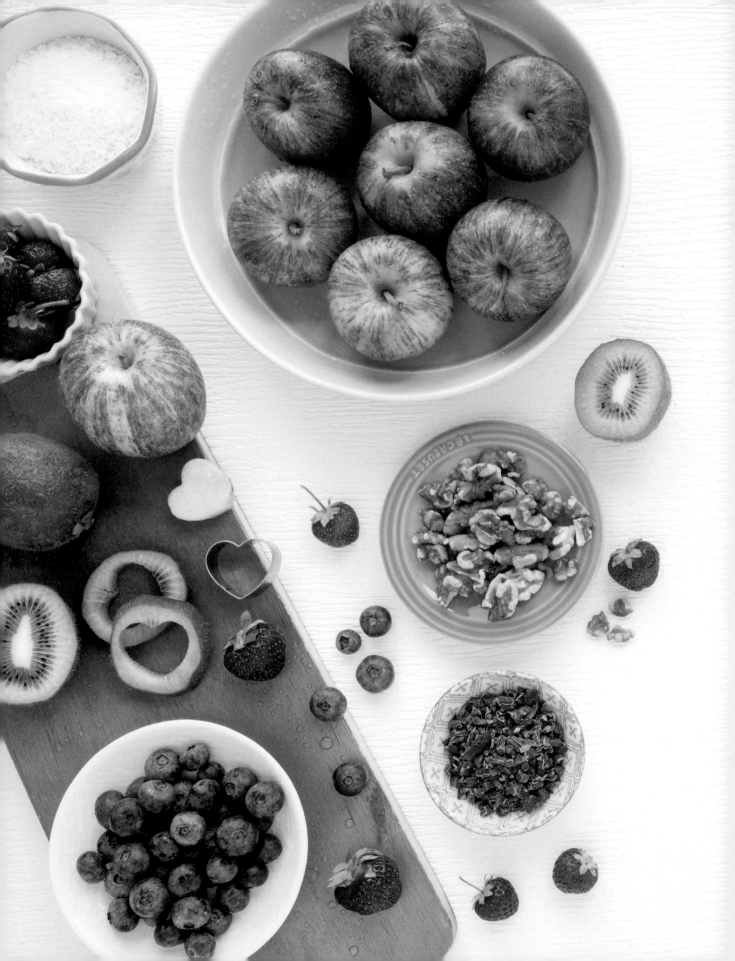

Breakfast and Brunch

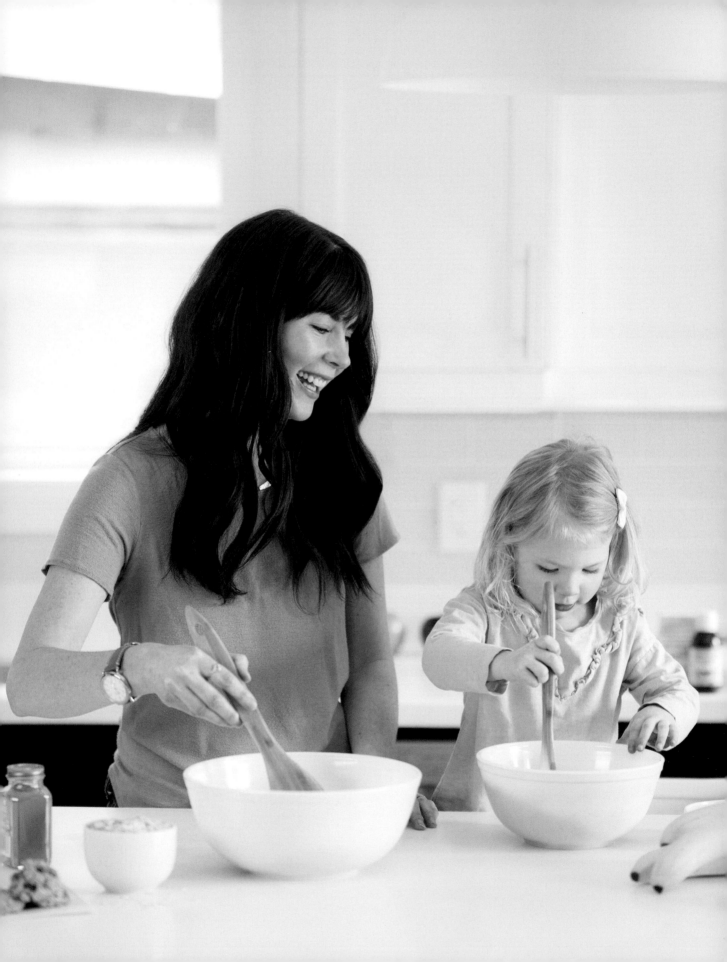

BREAKFAST AND BRUNCH

This might sound funny but I enjoy breakfast so much I think about it the night before when I go to bed. Not wanting to feel rushed in the morning, I always make sure we are up early enough to sit down to a healthy breakfast before the busyness of the day begins. Our day starts with a morning cuddle with Vienna. She sleeps in her own bed, but the second she is awake, she wants to snuggle in our bed. After cuddle time, we make breakfast. During the week our breakfast is quite simple. One day it might be a smoothie with Applesauce Spice Breakfast Muffins (page 18) or Oat Bran Cranberry Orange Two-Bite Muffins (page 21) that I made on the weekend, and another day it might be Best-Ever Granola (page 25) with coconut—healthy, yet simple and easy-to-make food.

Weekend mornings are definitely more leisurely because we usually don't have to be anywhere right away. We'll eat breakfast a little later, and often that turns into brunch. Walker loves savoury breakfasts like my Breakfast Buddha Bowl (page 41) or his Breakfast Sammie (page 38), while Vienna and I go for Stacked and Stuffed Blueberry Pancakes (page 26) or Apple Cinnamon Walnut Waffles (page 29). Vienna loves to help with the cooking, and it's fun to get messy in the kitchen when there's more time for play (and cleanup!). Weekends are made for leisure and slow food. But whether it's Sunday or Tuesday, mornings are my favourite time of the day. They are the perfect way to celebrate a brand-new day!

Applesauce Spice Breakfast Muffins
Dairy-free • Gluten-free • Grain-free • Kid-friendly • Vegetarian

Makes 6 muffins

Most of our mornings are fairly routine, but busy. My husband, Walker, and I get up by seven, wake up our daughter, Vienna (unless she's already awake), and have snuggle time, then make breakfast, get dressed, get her to school and get ourselves to the office. It's not usually hectic because we leave room for the routine, but there isn't a lot of time for leisure! That's why I make these muffins on a Sunday afternoon, so I'll have an extra ten or fifteen minutes of my morning back during the week.

These are super filling because of the protein and fibre in the coconut flour, yet fluffy, and they won't leave you feeling full or bloated. My favourite way to enjoy these muffins is to slice them in half and slather on some crunchy almond butter—heavenly! If I'm feeling like I need more, I will have a smoothie too, like my Green Mojito Smoothie (page 55). You can make a double batch of these muffins and freeze them. The consistency of baked goods made with coconut flour will change a bit when frozen, but they are still delicious!

Muffins
½ cup (125 mL) coconut flour
2 teaspoons (10 mL) baking powder
1 teaspoon (5 mL) cinnamon
1 teaspoon (5 mL) ground ginger
¼ teaspoon (1 mL) ground nutmeg
4 eggs
⅔ cup (150 mL) unsweetened applesauce
½ cup (125 mL) coconut oil, melted
¼ cup (60 mL) real maple syrup
2 teaspoons (10 mL) pure vanilla extract

Crumble Topping
2 tablespoons (30 mL) roughly chopped
  raw almonds
½ teaspoon (2 mL) cinnamon
½ teaspoon (2 mL) coconut sugar

1. **Make the Muffins** Preheat the oven to 350°F (180°C). Line a muffin tin with paper liners.

2. In a large bowl, stir together the coconut flour, baking powder, cinnamon, ginger and nutmeg.

3. In a small bowl, whisk the eggs, then whisk in the applesauce, coconut oil, maple syrup and vanilla. Add the wet mixture to the dry mixture and stir just until combined. Do not overmix. The batter will be very thick. Let the batter rest for 3 minutes.

4. **Meanwhile, make the Crumble Topping** In a small bowl, stir together the almonds, cinnamon and coconut sugar.

5. Spoon the batter evenly into the muffin cups. Top each muffin with the crumble. Bake for 30 to 35 minutes, until the tops are golden or a fork inserted in the centre of a muffin comes out clean. Be careful not to burn the muffins.

6. Let cool slightly in the tin and then transfer the muffins to a rack to cool completely before storing. Store in an airtight container in the fridge for up to 5 days or in the freezer for up to 3 months.

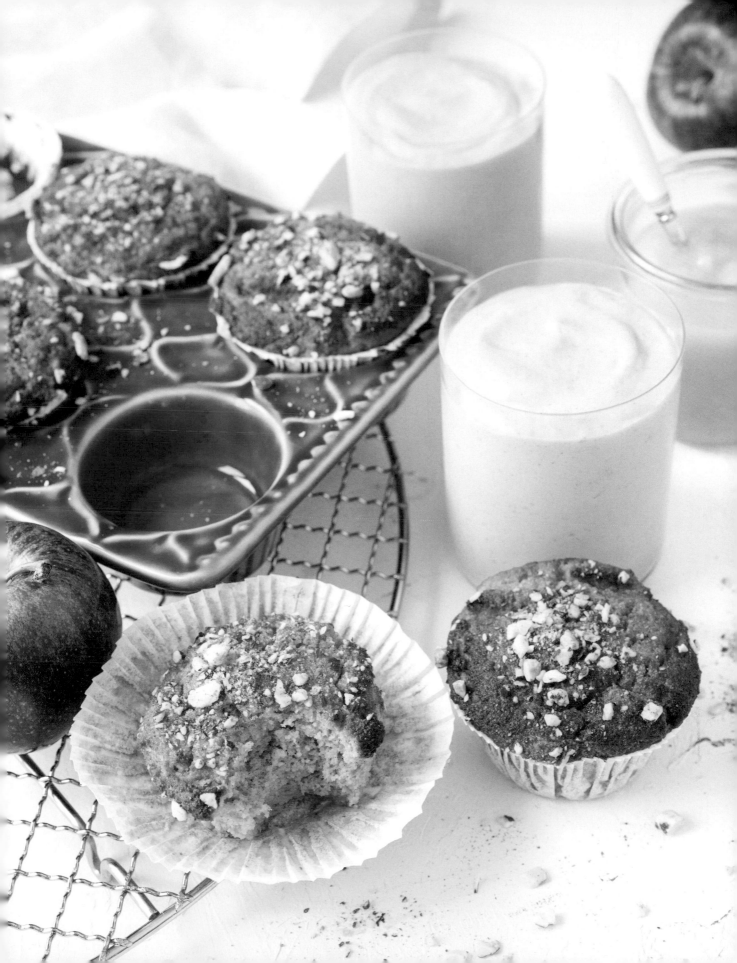

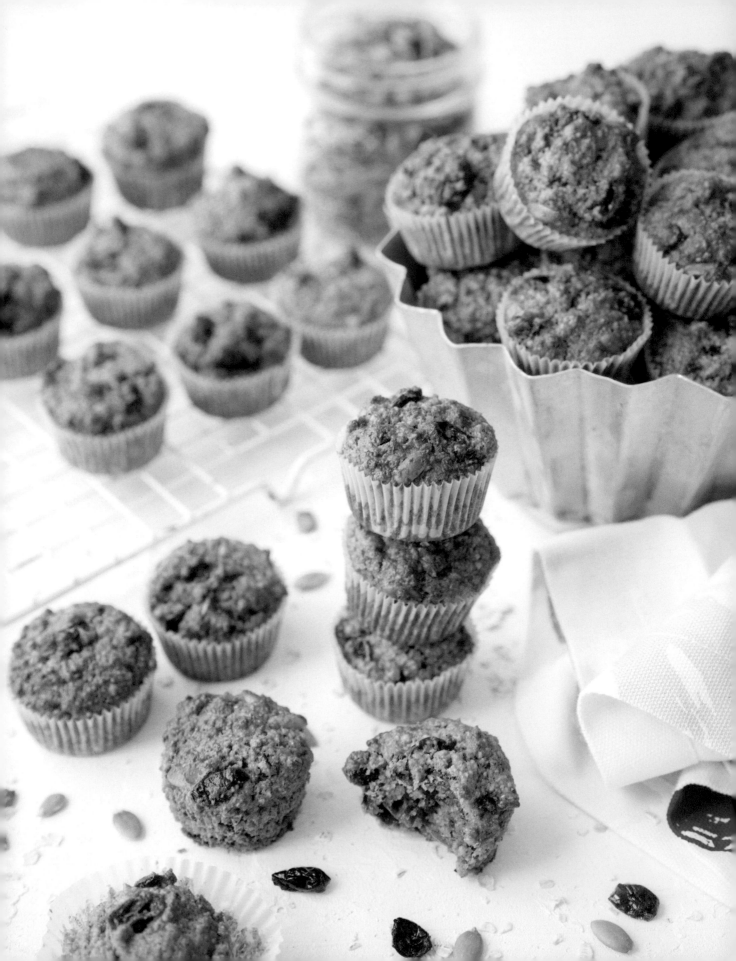

Oat Bran Cranberry Orange Two-Bite Muffins

Dairy-free • Kid-friendly • Vegetarian

Makes 24 mini muffins

I find that regular-size muffins often get wasted by my young daughter, smashed and pulled apart but not completely eaten, so I started making them bite-size, or in her case, a few bites. It worked! She loves these muffins because not only are they the perfect size but the orange zest and cranberries are a wonderful flavour match. Walker eats three or four of them at a time, so everyone is happy!

Oat bran is the nutrition star in these muffins. I feel most people overlook this superfood. It has a lot of soluble fibre, which absorbs nearly twenty-five times its weight in liquid, so it really fills you up and keeps you satisfied. Soluble fibre helps to slow the release of glucose into the blood stream so it's great for blood sugar control too. These muffins freeze really well as long as you put them in a freezer bag or wrap them well.

1 cup (250 mL) oat bran
¾ cup (175 mL) almond flour
  (almond meal)
¼ cup (60 mL) ground flaxseed (flax meal)
1 teaspoon (5 mL) baking soda
1 teaspoon (5 mL) cinnamon
½ teaspoon (2 mL) ground nutmeg
2 eggs
½ cup (125 mL) unsweetened almond milk
⅓ cup (75 mL) real maple syrup
2 tablespoons (30 mL) coconut oil, melted
1 to 2 tablespoons (15 to 30 mL) orange
  zest
1 cup (250 mL) dried cranberries
¼ cup (60 mL) raw pumpkin seeds

1. Position the oven racks in the top third and lower third of the oven and preheat the oven to 350°F (180°C). Line 2 mini muffin tins with paper liners or grease with coconut oil.

2. In a large bowl, stir together the oat bran, almond flour, flaxseed, baking soda, cinnamon and nutmeg.

3. In a small bowl, whisk the eggs, then whisk in the almond milk, maple syrup, coconut oil and orange zest. Add the wet mixture to the dry mixture and stir just until combined. Do not overmix. Fold in the cranberries and pumpkin seeds.

4. Spoon the batter evenly into the muffin cups. Bake for 15 to 20 minutes, until a fork inserted in the centre of a muffin comes out clean.

5. Let cool slightly in the tins and then turn the muffins out onto a rack to cool completely before storing. Store in an airtight container in the fridge for up to 5 days or in the freezer for up to 3 months.

Zucchini Blueberry Loaf

Dairy-free • Gluten-free • Kid-friendly • Nut-free • Vegetarian

Makes 1 loaf

I make a lot of muffins, but sometimes when life gets busy I just pour the batter into a loaf pan, pop it in the oven, and then I have about an hour to fold laundry or vacuum or just relax with a cup of tea. This loaf is filling and absolutely delicious thanks to the coconut flour, which is rich in fibre, protein and healthy fats. It's one of my favourite flours to use because it is full of goodness and it's darn tasty. (It's not a true flour in the traditional sense because it's made from dried and ground coconut meat.)

Consider yourself warned, though: this loaf will not last long. Once Walker and Vienna find out I've baked one of these, they polish it off in a day or two. After making this recipe, you can use the rest of your coconut flour to make my Applesauce Spice Breakfast Muffins (page 18). If you prefer to make muffins after all, bake them for 28 minutes.

½ cup (125 mL) grated zucchini
1 cup (250 mL) fresh or thawed frozen blueberries
1 ripe banana, mashed
2 eggs, beaten
½ cup (125 mL) dark real maple syrup (I use No. 3)
¼ cup (60 mL) coconut oil, melted
¼ cup (60 mL) unsweetened non-dairy milk (rice or coconut milk)
¼ cup (60 mL) unsweetened applesauce
1 teaspoon (5 mL) pure vanilla extract
1 cup (250 mL) brown rice flour
½ cup (125 mL) coconut flour
1 teaspoon (5 mL) baking powder
1 teaspoon (5 mL) baking soda
1 teaspoon (5 mL) cinnamon
½ teaspoon (2 mL) ground nutmeg

1. Preheat the oven to 350°F (180°C). Line the bottom and sides of an 8½- × 4½-inch (1.5 L) loaf pan with parchment paper or grease generously with coconut oil. If using a muffin tin, line with paper liners or grease with coconut oil.

2. Place the grated zucchini in a fine-mesh strainer or nut milk bag and press or wring out excess water. Don't skip this step or your loaf will be too wet.

3. In a large bowl, stir together the zucchini, blueberries, banana, beaten eggs, maple syrup, coconut oil, applesauce, non-dairy milk and vanilla.

4. In another large bowl, stir together the brown rice flour, coconut flour, baking powder, baking soda, cinnamon and nutmeg. Add the wet mixture to the dry mixture and stir just until combined. Do not overmix. The batter will be very thick.

5. Scrape the batter into the pan and smooth the top. Bake for 50 to 60 minutes, until a knife inserted in the centre of the loaf comes out clean. If the top starts to brown before it's fully cooked, cover the top loosely with foil.

6. Let cool in the pan for 10 minutes before turning the loaf out onto a rack. Let cool for at least 10 more minutes before slicing. Store in an airtight container in the fridge for up to 1 week or slice, wrap individually and freeze in a resealable plastic freezer bag for up to 3 months.

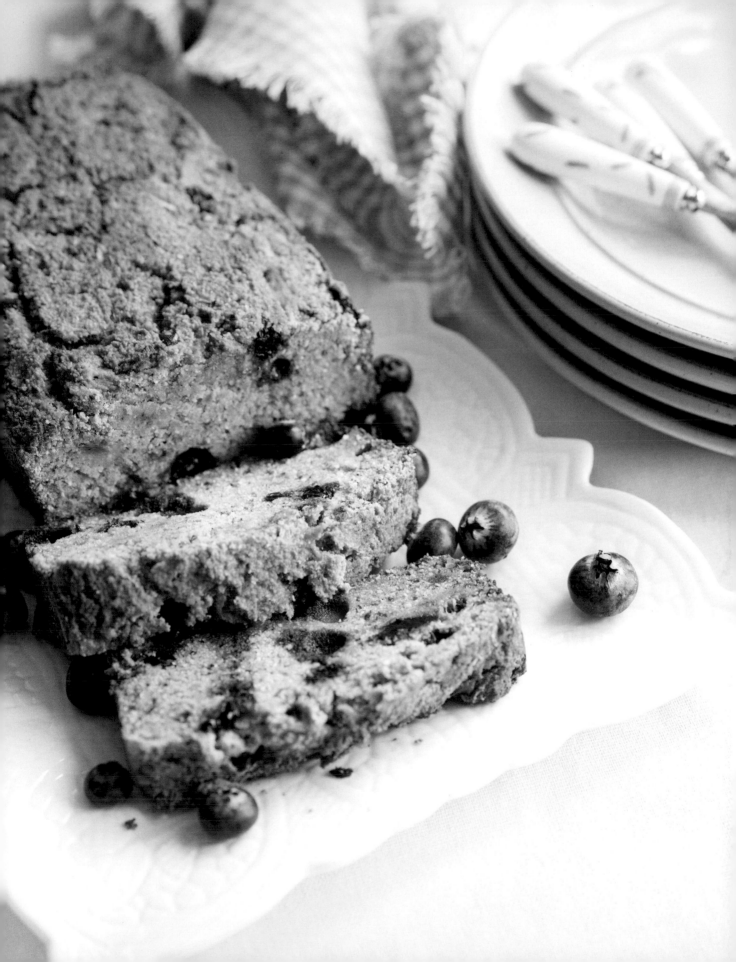

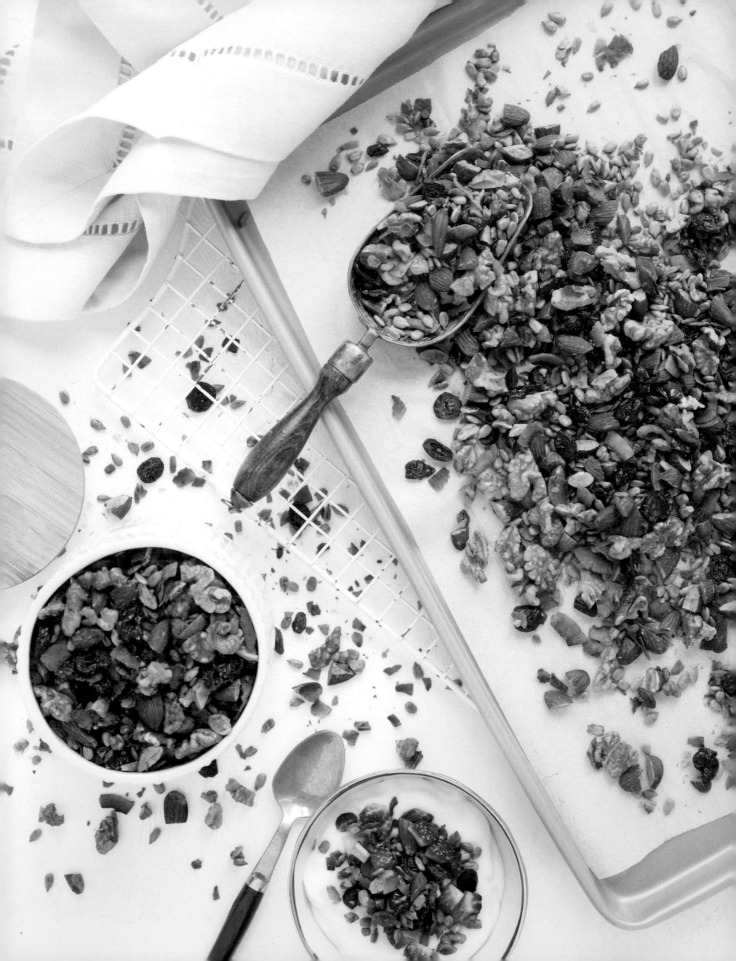

Best-Ever Granola

Dairy-free • Gluten-free • Grain-free • Kid-friendly • Vegan

Makes 6½ cups (1.75 L)

If you've ever made your own granola at home, you've probably said to yourself, *Why would I ever buy granola again? This is the best!* Homemade granola is not only very easy to make, but it's free from all the refined sugar and additives you often find in store-bought varieties—and it tastes amazing. You get to decide what the ingredients will be. The best part of making your own is the smell while it's baking. That is reason enough to make it yourself.

   Sometimes when hunger strikes and it's not mealtime, I just grab a handful of this to tide me over. My favourite way to enjoy it, though, is mixed in with some coconut or sheep's milk yogurt and fresh fruit. When you're baking the granola, be sure not to overcrowd the baking sheet or it won't toast evenly.

2 cups (500 mL) chopped raw almonds
2 cups (500 mL) chopped raw walnuts
1 cup (250 mL) raw sunflower seeds
1 cup (250 mL) unsweetened coconut flakes
½ cup (125 mL) unsweetened dried
   blueberries or cranberries
¼ cup (60 mL) coconut oil
¼ cup (60 mL) real maple syrup
1 teaspoon (5 mL) cinnamon
1 teaspoon (5 mL) ground ginger
½ teaspoon (2 mL) ground cardamom
½ teaspoon (2 mL) sea salt

1. Position the oven racks in the top third and lower third of the oven and preheat the oven to 350°F (180°C). Line 2 baking sheets with parchment paper or grease well with coconut oil.

2. In a large bowl, combine the almonds, walnuts, sunflower seeds, coconut flakes and blueberries.

3. In a small pot, melt the coconut oil over low heat. Stir in the maple syrup, cinnamon, ginger, cardamom and sea salt. Add the coconut oil mixture to the nut mixture and stir to combine well.

4. Divide the mixture between the prepared baking sheets, spreading it evenly and making sure not to overcrowd the pans. Bake for 10 to 15 minutes or until it starts to brown. Stir the granola, then bake for another 5 to 10 minutes, until golden brown. Be careful not to let the granola burn.

5. Let cool completely on the baking sheets. Transfer to an airtight container, preferably a mason jar, and store at room temperature for up to 4 weeks.

Stacked and Stuffed Blueberry Pancakes

Dairy-free • Kid-friendly • Vegetarian

Makes 12 pancakes

Weekends call for pancakes, and if you read my blog, *Joyous Health*, you probably know I'm a pancake monster. The ingredients I use have evolved over the years, so I'm happy to report that these pancakes will leave you with zero food guilt because they are super healthy, they're packed with wholesome real ingredients and they'll keep your belly joyous for hours. They might look intimidating, but they are simply pancakes stacked on top of each other with a fruit stuffing in between—super easy! But you don't have to stack and stuff them—the pancakes are delicious all on their own.

If you're having trouble finding oat flour, you can blitz 2 cups (500 mL) oat flakes or old-fashioned rolled oats in a mini food processor until you've made flour. You can mix the batter in a mixing bowl, but I prefer to use the food processor so the blueberries become part of the batter—the colour is part of this recipe's magic.

Blueberry Chia Seed Jam
2 cups (500 mL) fresh or thawed frozen
  blueberries
2 tablespoons (30 mL) chia seeds
½ teaspoon (2 mL) cinnamon
1 tablespoon (15 mL) coconut sugar
  (optional)

Blueberry Pancakes
2 cups (500 mL) oat flour
2 tablespoons (30 mL) ground flaxseed
  (flax meal)
2 ripe bananas, mashed
2 eggs
1 cup (250 mL) fresh or thawed frozen
  blueberries
1 cup (250 mL) unsweetened almond milk
1 tablespoon (15 mL) coconut oil, for frying

Stuffing and Toppings
¼ cup (60 mL) coconut butter
½ cup (125 mL) chopped fresh strawberries
½ cup (125 mL) fresh blueberries
2 ripe bananas, sliced
¼ cup (60 mL) real maple syrup

1. **Make the Blueberry Chia Seed Jam** Combine the blueberries, chia seeds and cinnamon in a food processor and process until chunky. If the blueberries are not sweet, add the coconut sugar. If you're not using the jam right away, transfer it to a mason jar and store in the fridge for up to 1 week.

2. **Make the Blueberry Pancakes** Preheat the oven to 200°F (100°C). Line a baking sheet with parchment paper.

3. Wipe the bowl of the food processor clean. Combine the oat flour, flaxseed, bananas, eggs, blueberries and almond milk. Process until smooth. The batter will be very thick.

4. In a large frying pan, heat the coconut oil over medium heat. Make sure the pan is hot before adding any pancake batter. Add ¼ cup (60 mL) of batter for each pancake. Cook for 3 minutes. (You probably won't see bubbles.) Flip and cook for 2 to 3 more minutes, until golden brown on the bottom. Transfer to the prepared baking sheet and keep warm in the oven while you cook the remaining pancakes.

5. In a small pot, slowly melt the coconut butter over low heat. Be careful because it burns very easily.

6. To serve, place a pancake on a plate and top with some chia jam. Place another pancake on top and spread with some melted coconut butter. Repeat to make a stack as high as you like. Top with strawberries, blueberries and sliced banana and drizzle with maple syrup.

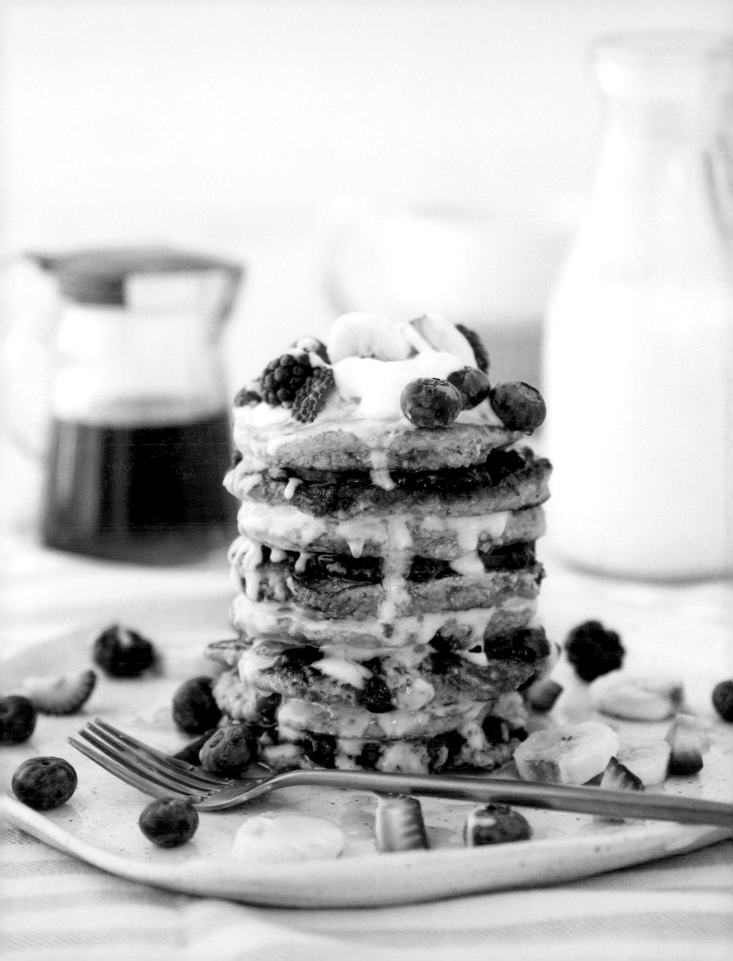

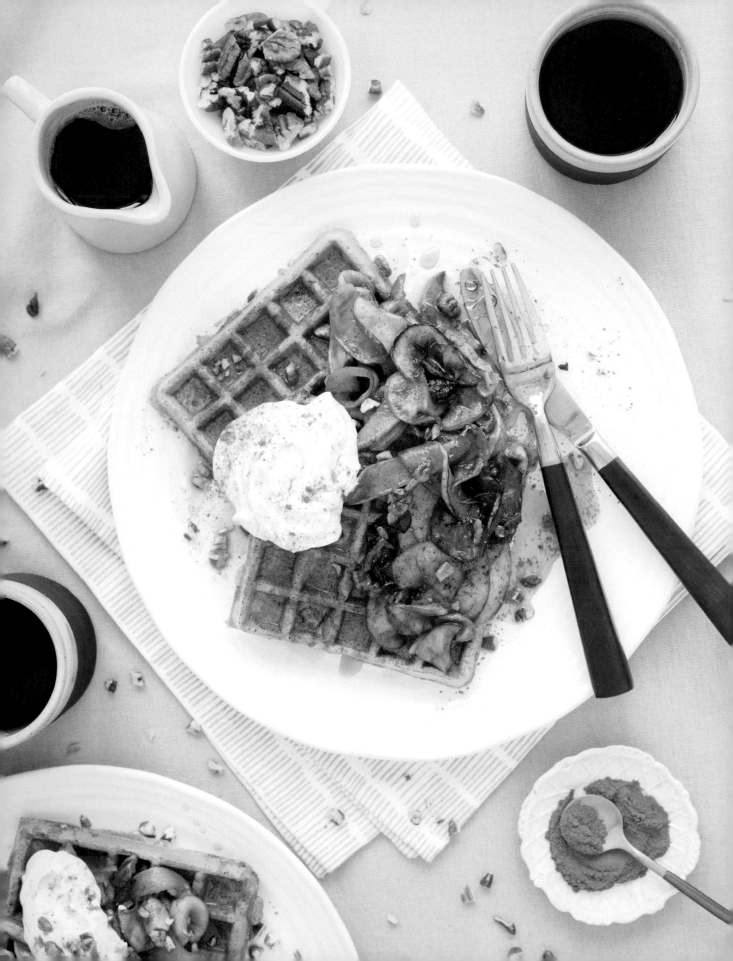

Apple Cinnamon Walnut Waffles

Dairy-free • Gluten-free • Kid-friendly • Vegetarian

Makes 12 waffles

Warmed apples with walnuts and maple syrup make these waffles perfect for weekend brunch, especially when it's chilly outside. I didn't grow up eating waffles—we were a pancake family—but for as long as I can remember I've wanted a waffle iron. One day I took the plunge, and it was worth every penny. Waffles are just so satisfying—golden and crunchy on the outside and fluffy and warm on the inside.

Most glutinous flours will work in this recipe, but buckwheat flour is my go-to gluten-free flour for pancakes, so it only made sense to include it in my waffle recipe. Spelt or kamut flour work as well.

Apple Cinnamon Waffles

1½ cups (375 mL) light buckwheat flour
2 teaspoons (10 mL) baking powder
1 teaspoon (5 mL) cinnamon
2 eggs
¼ cup (60 mL) unsweetened almond milk
½ cup (125 mL) unsweetened applesauce

Apple Walnut Topping

1 tablespoon (15 mL) coconut oil
1 apple (Royal Gala or McIntosh),
  thinly sliced
¼ cup (60 mL) chopped raw walnuts
2 tablespoons (30 mL) real maple syrup
½ teaspoon (2 mL) cinnamon
Plain full-fat coconut yogurt, for serving

1. Preheat the waffle iron. Preheat the oven to 200°F (100°C) and line a baking sheet with parchment paper.

2. **Make the waffle batter** In a large bowl, whisk together the buckwheat flour, baking powder and cinnamon.

3. In a small bowl, whisk the eggs, then whisk in the almond milk and applesauce. Add the wet mixture to the dry mixture and stir until combined.

4. **Make the Apple Walnut Topping** In a small saucepan, melt the coconut oil over medium heat. Stir in the sliced apples and cook, stirring occasionally, for 4 to 5 minutes, until fork-tender. Stir in the walnuts, maple syrup and cinnamon. Remove from the heat and cover with a lid to keep warm until serving.

5. Meanwhile, if necessary, grease the waffle iron with coconut oil. Ladle about ⅓ cup (75 mL) of the waffle batter into the waffle iron, spreading it to the edges. Cook the waffles until golden and crisp, 4 to 5 minutes. Transfer waffles to the prepared baking sheet and keep warm in the oven while you cook the remaining waffles.

6. To serve, top each waffle with warm Apple Walnut Topping and a spoonful of coconut yogurt.

Peachy Parfait with Peach Chia Seed Jam

Gluten-free • Grain-free • Kid-friendly • Vegetarian

Makes 4 parfaits

I love when peaches are in season—they are perfectly sweet and so juicy. If you're making this when peaches are not in season, you can use thawed frozen peach slices. Peaches are very rich in antioxidants that fight oxidative stress. One particular antioxidant, caffeic acid, is especially high in peaches and it protects the body from a mould commonly found in peanuts, almonds and corn.

    The two types of yogurt I use most often are plain coconut yogurt and sheep's milk yogurt. Either will work in these parfaits. Another wonderful option is kefir, which is rich in friendly bacteria, making it ideal for good digestion. Even though most kefir is made with cow's milk, you can find coconut kefir in some health food stores. I suggest making the peach jam ahead of time. It freezes well, and if you make a large batch when peaches are in season, you'll be able to enjoy peach jam for many months.

Peach Chia Seed Jam

2 cups (500 mL) fresh or thawed frozen peaches
1 tablespoon (15 mL) chia seeds
1 tablespoon (15 mL) pure liquid honey (optional)

Peachy Parfait

2 cups (500 mL) Best-Ever Granola (page 25)
1 cup (250 mL) sliced fresh peaches
2 cups (500 mL) unsweetened plain full-fat yogurt
1 cup (250 mL) Peach Chia Seed Jam (recipe above)

1. **Make the Peach Chia Seed Jam** Combine the peaches, chia seeds and honey, if using, in a food processor and blend until smooth. Transfer to an airtight container and refrigerate overnight before using. The jam will keep in the fridge for up to 1 week or in the freezer for up to 3 months.

2. **Make the Peach Parfait** Spoon 2 tablespoons (30 mL) of Best-Ever Granola into 4 medium glasses. Add some of the peach slices, then a large dollop of yogurt, and top with a dollop of Peach Chia Seed Jam. Repeat layers 2 or 3 times, until the glasses are full. Top with sliced peaches.

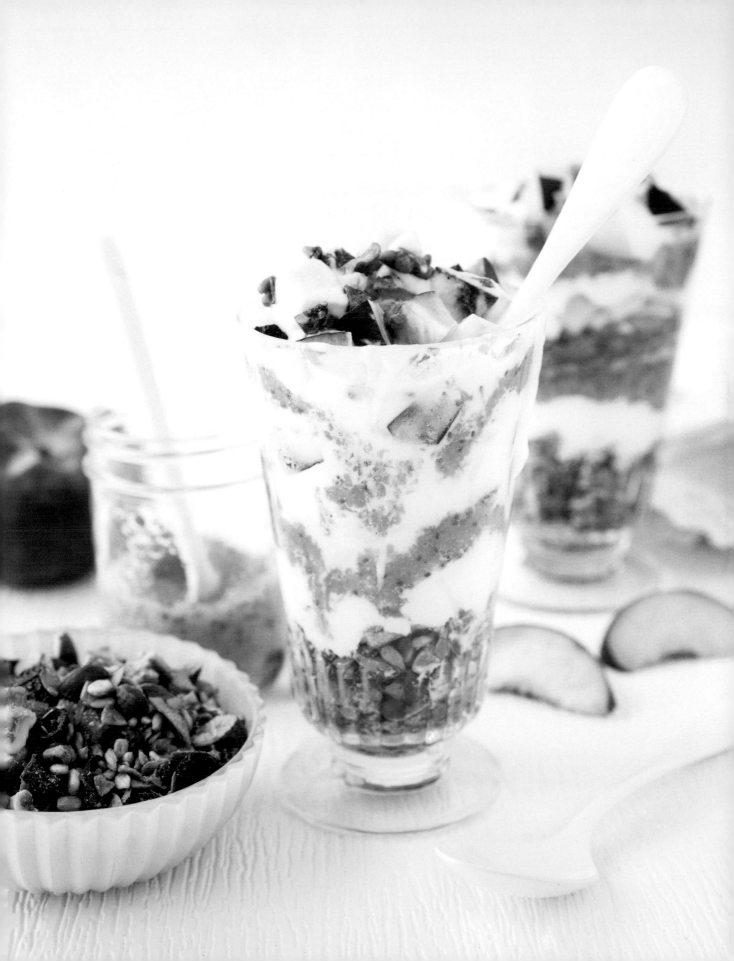

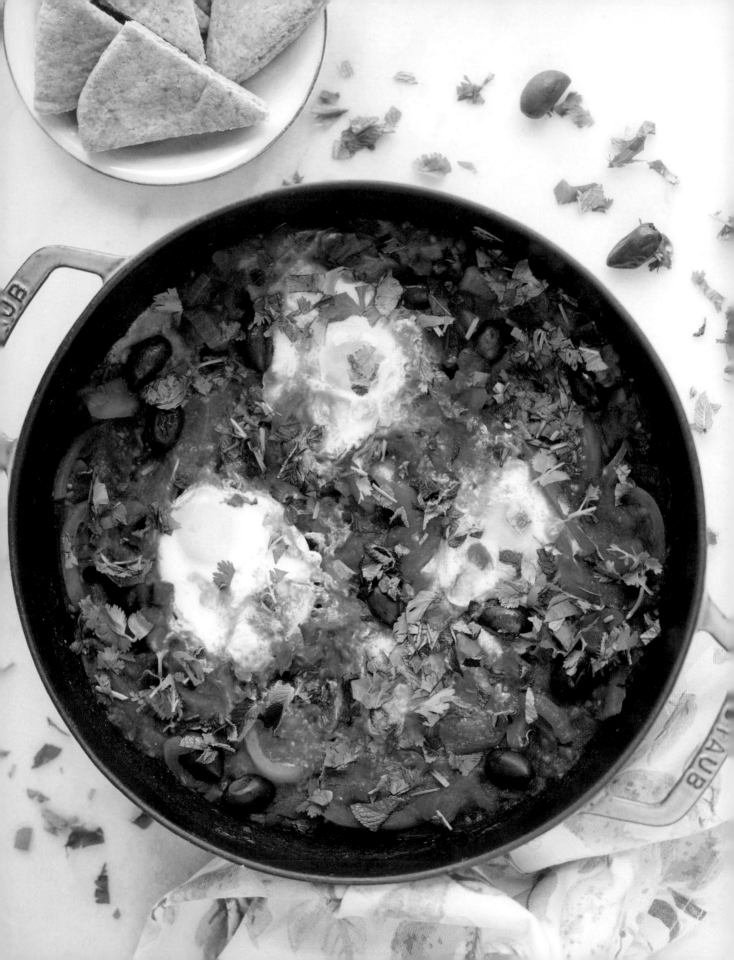

Shakshuka

Dairy-free • Gluten-free • Grain-free • Nut-free • Vegetarian

Serves 4

Even though I'd been eating eggs in tomato sauce for years, I never knew it was called shakshuka and originated in northern Africa. It became huge in Israel and is now a super-popular brunch dish in many countries. We discovered it at a restaurant in Toronto. It became one of those dishes that we often ordered when out for brunch but never made at home. I decided to take the plunge and discovered that it's very easy to make.

This dish is an absolute hit if you're hosting brunch because, really, who doesn't love eggs with tomatoes? The best part about this recipe is you probably have all the ingredients in your kitchen already, and if you don't, they are no further than your nearest grocery store.

1 tablespoon (15 mL) extra-virgin olive oil
½ red onion, thinly sliced
3 cloves garlic, finely chopped
1 sweet yellow pepper, thinly sliced
1 sweet orange pepper, thinly sliced
1 teaspoon (5 mL) sweet paprika
½ teaspoon (2 mL) cayenne pepper
½ teaspoon (2 mL) ground cumin
8 medium vine-ripened tomatoes, chopped
4 eggs
2 tablespoons (30 mL) chopped fresh mint,
 for garnish
2 tablespoons (30 mL) chopped fresh
 cilantro, for garnish
Pita bread or Za'atar Socca (page 130),
 for serving

1. In a large frying pan (I like using a braiser), heat the olive oil over medium heat. Add the red onion and cook, stirring occasionally, until soft and translucent, about 5 minutes. Add the garlic and sweet peppers and cook, stirring occasionally, for 2 minutes. Add the paprika, cayenne and cumin; cook, stirring occasionally, for 2 more minutes. Stir in the tomatoes and simmer for 10 to 15 minutes until fragrant and the tomatoes have softened. If the sauce starts to dry out, add 1 to 2 tablespoons (15 to 30 mL) water.

2. Using a spoon, create 4 wells in the tomato sauce. Gently crack an egg into each well. Reduce the heat to low, cover the pan with a lid and cook until the egg whites are set but the yolks are still runny.

3. Sprinkle the mint and cilantro on top and serve immediately with pita bread or socca.

Sweet Potato and Spinach Mini Frittatas

Gluten-free • Grain-free • Kid-friendly • Vegetarian

Makes 16 mini frittatas

When entertaining family and friends on weekends, frittatas are my go-to—always a crowd-pleaser and so easy to put together. I often cook the sweet potato the day before so I've got that out of the way, especially if I'm making other dishes to go along with the frittatas. I like making mini frittatas because they are fun and portable—that's a good enough reason, isn't it? But, if you want to make this even easier for yourself, skip the muffin tins and bake the whole frittata in a lasagna pan.

You could use butternut squash in place of the sweet potato for a nice change. If you're lucky enough to have leftovers, have a mini frittata for lunch the next day with a big salad like my Broccoli and Cranberry Salad with Creamy Dill Dressing (page 104). You can reheat these in the oven at 350°F (180°C) for 10 minutes or eat them chilled.

2 cups (500 mL) sweet potato, cut into small cubes
2 tablespoons (30 mL) extra-virgin olive oil, divided
Pinch of sea salt
1 medium white onion, finely chopped
12 eggs
½ cup (125 mL) unsweetened almond milk or your favourite nut milk
1 teaspoon (5 mL) Italian seasoning
1 teaspoon (5 mL) garlic powder
1 cup (250 mL) chopped fresh spinach
½ cup (125 mL) crumbled feta cheese

1. Preheat the oven to 350°F (180°C). Line a baking sheet with parchment paper. Grease a mini muffin tin or 13- × 9-inch (3.5 L) lasagna pan with coconut oil.

2. Spread the sweet potatoes on the prepared baking sheet. Toss with 1 tablespoon (15 mL) of the olive oil and sprinkle with sea salt. Bake for 35 to 40 minutes, until fork-tender. Let the sweet potatoes cool slightly.

3. In a medium frying pan, heat the remaining 1 tablespoon (15 mL) olive oil over medium heat. Add the onion and cook, stirring occasionally, until soft and translucent, about 5 minutes. Remove from the heat.

4. In a large bowl, whisk together the eggs, almond milk, Italian seasoning and garlic powder. Stir in the spinach, feta, onions and baked sweet potato.

5. Fill the muffin cups about three-quarters full. Bake for 15 to 20 minutes, until the frittatas have risen and are golden on top. If using a lasagna pan, bake for 30 to 35 minutes.

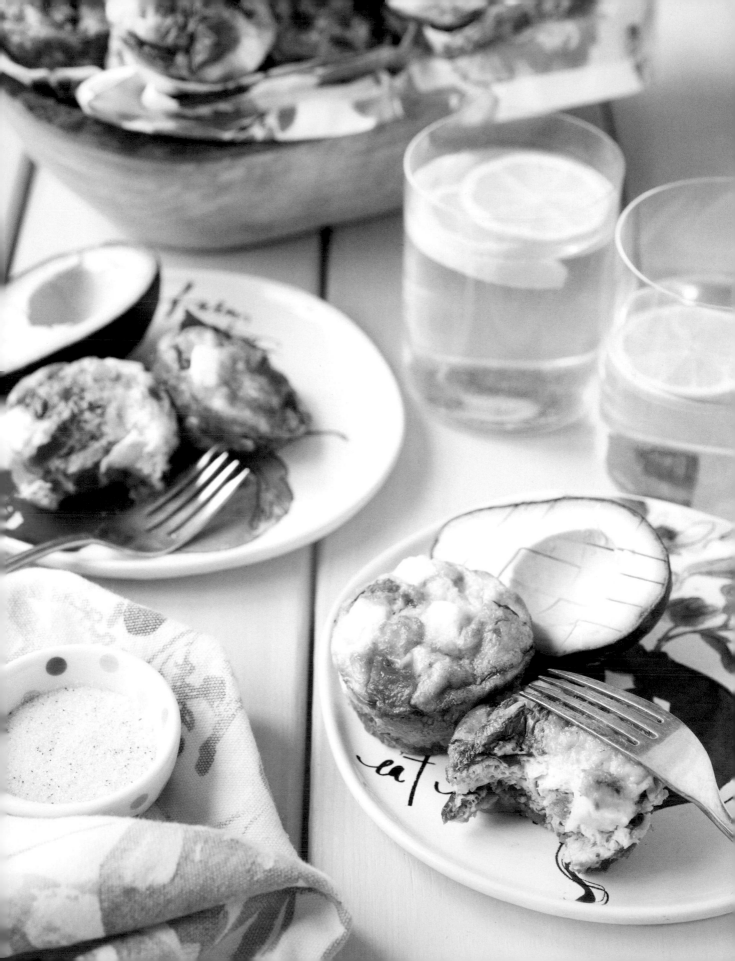

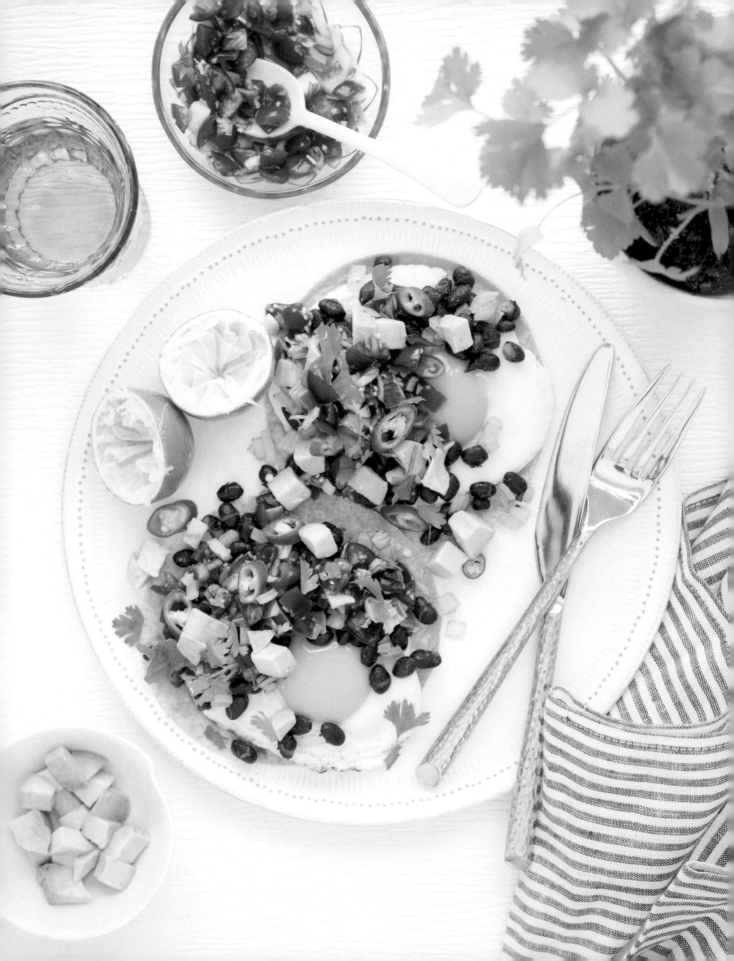

Breakfast Tacos with Salsa

Gluten-free • Kid-friendly • Nut-free • Vegetarian

Makes 6 tacos

Tacos are a good idea any time of year—or any time of day! I honestly can't think of any reason not to make them. But the funny thing is, tacos for a long time were something I only ate at restaurants or drooled over on Instagram. One day, after realizing I'd saved at least thirty-five different #tacotuesday photos to my phone, I decided to make them myself. What a joyous idea! They are so easy and you can't screw them up!

These breakfast tacos are super balanced. They have protein from the eggs and beans, good fats from the avocado and egg yolk, pops of flavour and heat, and lots of fibre. This is the perfect recipe for feeling fabulous for the whole dang day! You could use whatever tortilla shell you prefer. I like both corn tortillas and raw tortillas made from vegetables and flax seeds, which you can usually find at your local health food store. And if you're like me and you prefer scrambled eggs, you can do that too.

Salsa
4 cups (1 L) grape tomatoes, chopped
2 jalapeño peppers or Thai green chili peppers, seeded and finely chopped
2 cloves garlic, minced
1 small red onion, finely chopped
¼ cup (60 mL) finely chopped fresh cilantro
Juice of 1 lime

Breakfast Tacos
1 tablespoon (15 mL) extra-virgin olive oil
1 small white onion, chopped
1 clove garlic, chopped
½ teaspoon (2 mL) ground cumin
1 can (14 ounces/398 mL) black beans, drained and rinsed
1 tablespoon (15 mL) Original Ghee (page 43), store-bought ghee or unsalted butter
6 eggs
6 small corn tortillas
2 ripe avocados, pitted, peeled and cubed
¼ cup (60 mL) loosely packed chopped fresh cilantro
Hot sauce (optional)

1. **Make the Salsa** In a small bowl, combine the tomatoes, jalapeños, garlic, red onion, cilantro and lime juice. Stir well. Set aside.

2. **Make the Breakfast Tacos** In a large frying pan, heat the olive oil over medium heat. Add the onion and cook, stirring occasionally, until soft and translucent, about 5 minutes. Stir in the garlic, cumin and black beans and cook until the beans are heated through. Transfer the mixture to a bowl.

3. Wipe the pan clean, then add the Original Ghee and melt over medium-high heat. Break the eggs into the pan and cook until the whites are set, 4 to 5 minutes.

4. To assemble, place an egg on each corn tortilla and top with the black bean mixture, avocado, cilantro, Salsa and hot sauce to taste, if using.

Walker's Breakfast Sammie

Nut-free

Serves 2

In our home we call sandwiches sammies. Since my husband, Walker, loves his sammies, I knew we had to put at least one in this cookbook. I've never been much of a sandwich person, but I always steal a bite or two of Walker's because they are so yummy. His sammies pack as many simple ingredients as you could possibly imagine between two slices of bread, but everything combines in a delicious feast of flavours.

   If pork or bacon is not your thing, you can thinly slice some tempeh and pan-grill it for that meaty texture. It is just as delicious. My Turmeric Ghee adds a burst of flavour to the eggs, and the Quick Pickled Onions have that perfect level of tanginess this sammie calls for. I won't sugar-coat it: you may need a nap after this sammie. It's pretty filling!

4 slices of organic bacon
1 tablespoon (15 mL) Turmeric Ghee
   (page 44) or store-bought ghee
2 eggs
Pinch of sea salt
4 slices of buckwheat sourdough bread,
   toasted
2 teaspoons (10 mL) maple Dijon mustard
4 slices of tomato
½ ripe avocado, pitted, peeled and sliced
¼ cup (60 mL) Quick Pickled Onions
   (page 133)
Broccoli sprouts or pea sprouts
¼ cup (60 mL) grated Parmesan cheese

1. In a large frying pan over medium heat, cook the bacon until crispy, about 10 minutes.

2. When the bacon is about half-cooked, in a medium frying pan, melt the Turmeric Ghee over medium-high heat. Crack the eggs into the pan and cook until the whites are set, 4 to 5 minutes. Remove from the heat and sprinkle with sea salt.

3. To assemble, spread the mustard on 2 pieces of toasted sourdough bread. Top each of the 2 remaining slices with half of the bacon, tomatoes, avocado, Quick Pickled Onions, an egg, broccoli sprouts and Parmesan. Close the sandwiches and enjoy right away.

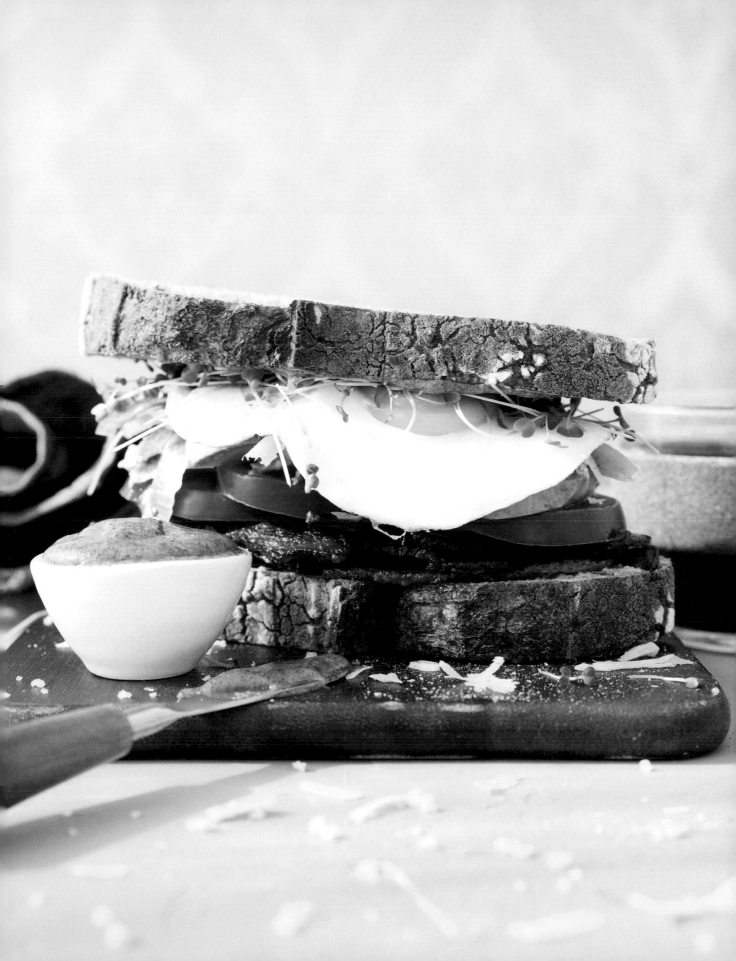

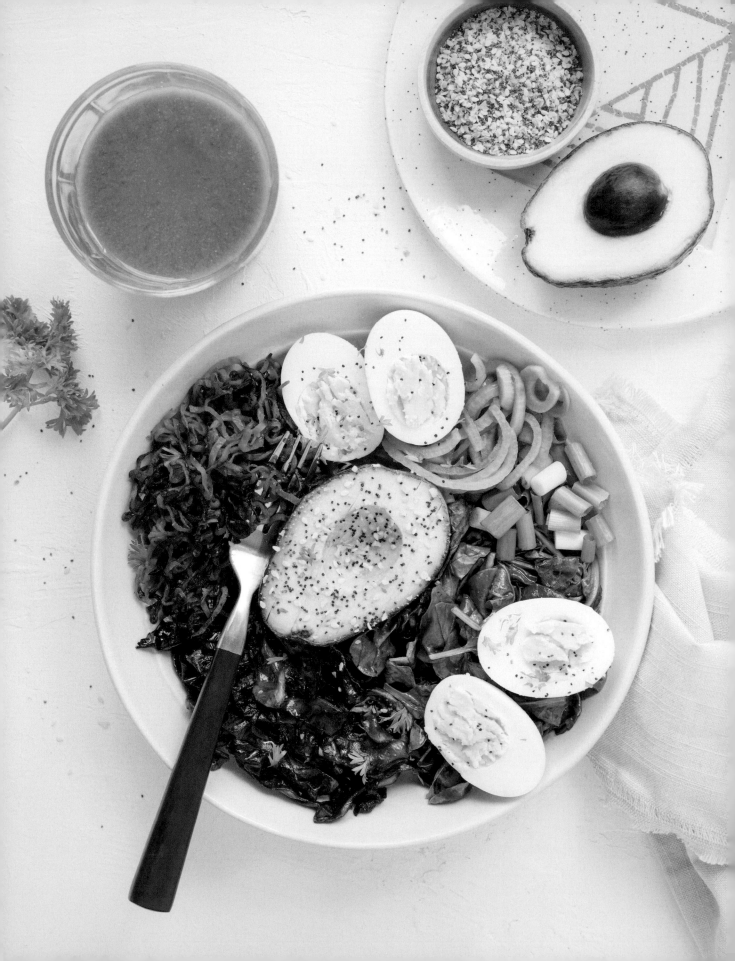

Breakfast Buddha Bowl

Gluten-free • Grain-free • Nut-free • Vegetarian

Serves 4

After a busy week, I crave meals like this on the weekend when we can slow down. The comfort of a home-cooked breakfast makes me forget any stresses from the week. There is no formula for the perfect Buddha bowl—you just put all your favourite ingredients together in a bowl and voila. I absolutely love including warmed cabbage in cooler months, but in the summer I use sauerkraut instead. Spiralizing sweet potato takes a bit of work, but it's well worth the few extra minutes. Don't worry if you don't have a spiralizer: you can just grate or finely chop the sweet potato instead.

Once a month, I make a batch of Avocado Sprinkle because it adds a nice texture and a hit of taste to whatever you sprinkle it on. It works on everything from baked sweet potatoes to avocado toast. Store it in an airtight container at room temperature for up to 3 months.

Avocado Sprinkle

2 tablespoons (30 mL) chia seeds
2 teaspoons (10 mL) sesame seeds
2 tablespoons (30 mL) onion flakes
2 teaspoons (10 mL) garlic powder

Buddha Bowl

2 tablespoons (30 mL) Original Ghee
    (page 43), store-bought ghee or
    extra-virgin olive oil
2 sweet potatoes, spiralized
½ purple cabbage, thinly sliced
    (or ½ cup/125 mL sauerkraut)
1 teaspoon (5 mL) dried rosemary
½ teaspoon (2 mL) sea salt, more to taste
Pepper
2 cups (500 mL) chopped fresh spinach
8 eggs
2 ripe avocados, pitted, peeled and cut
    in half
4 green onions (white and light green
    parts only), chopped
½ cup (125 mL) Quick Pickled Onions
    (page 133)
2 tablespoons (30 mL) chopped fresh
    curly or flat-leaf parsley

1. **Make the Avocado Sprinkle** In a small bowl, stir together the chia seeds, sesame seeds, onion flakes and garlic powder.

2. **Make the Buddha Bowl** In a medium frying pan, heat the Original Ghee over medium heat. Add the sweet potato and cabbage and cook, stirring occasionally, until the vegetables are soft but not mushy, about 5 minutes. Add the rosemary, sea salt and pepper to taste. Transfer the mixture to a bowl and set aside.

3. Return the pan (you don't need to wipe it clean) to medium heat, add the spinach and cook for 1 minute just to warm it. Remove from the heat and set aside.

4. To hard-boil the eggs, bring a large pot of water to a gentle boil with a pinch of sea salt. (The salt prevents the egg white from spreading in the water if the shell cracks.) Gently lower the eggs into the water and boil for 6 or 7 minutes. Drain the eggs and run under cold water. Peel the eggs and slice in half.

5. To assemble, in each of 4 large bowls like pasta bowls, place half an avocado in the middle. Top with the Avocado Sprinkle. Arrange the sweet potato mixture, spinach, green onions, Quick Pickled Onions and 4 hard-boiled egg halves around each avocado. Sprinkle with the parsley and sea salt to taste.

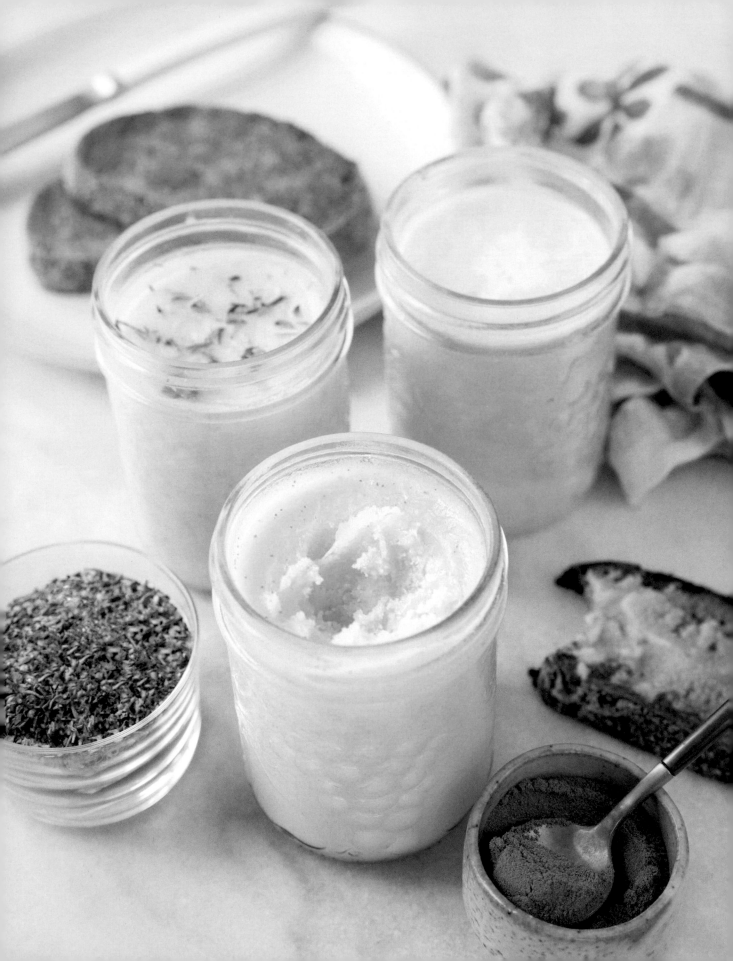

Ghee Three Ways

Each variation makes 1½ cups (375 mL)

I am in love with ghee. I started using it when I was in school studying nutrition, after hearing other students talk about how nutritious it is. After years of buying it, I realized it was more affordable to just make it! I prefer it to butter in most of my recipes because it has an incredibly rich flavour (a little goes a long way) and it has a high smoke point, making it perfect for cooking.

What exactly is ghee? It is butter that has been melted down and "clarified" to remove dairy proteins such as casein and whey, which are common allergens. Ghee is the next best thing when you can't enjoy butter! An important step that differentiates ghee from clarified butter is that once all the dairy proteins have been removed, you cook it a little longer, until you see browning on the bottom of the pot and the ghee becomes fragrant and more flavourful.

Making ghee is easy, but it does take some patience and time—it can take anywhere from 20 to 30 minutes from start to finish. I use it to make everything from pancakes to scrambled eggs to veggie stir-fries. It's delicious slathered on my Sun-Dried Tomato Olive Bread (page 82).

Original Ghee
Gluten-free • Grain-free • Nut-free • Vegetarian

1 pound (450 g) unsalted butter, cubed

1. Melt the butter in a medium pot, preferably with a heavy bottom so it doesn't easily burn, over medium heat. Once the butter melts, it will start to bubble and the milk proteins will begin to separate from the fat and float to the surface. Using a spoon, skim off these milk proteins. Reduce the heat to medium-low and continue cooking until the ghee is clear and you've skimmed off all the protein, 15 to 20 minutes.

2. Once it's clear, you have clarified butter, but to make ghee, continue to cook. In 5 to 10 more minutes, the milk solids that were not skimmed off will settle to the bottom of the pan and start to brown. Cook for 4 to 5 more minutes to enhance the richness of the flavour.

3. Remove from the heat and let the ghee cool for a few minutes. Pour it through cheesecloth or a fine-mesh strainer into a mason jar to strain out any remaining milk proteins. When the ghee is completely cool, seal with a lid. Store in the fridge for up to 6 months.

recipe continues

Turmeric Ghee
Gluten-free • Grain-free • Nut-free • Vegetarian

1 pound (450 g) unsalted butter, cubed
½ teaspoon (2 mL) ground turmeric

1. Melt the butter in a medium pot, preferably with a heavy bottom so it doesn't easily burn, over medium heat. Once the butter melts, it will start to bubble and the milk proteins will begin to separate from the fat and float to the surface. Using a spoon, skim off these milk proteins. Reduce the heat to medium-low and continue cooking until the ghee is clear and you've skimmed off all the protein, 15 to 20 minutes.

2. Once it's clear, you have clarified butter, but to make ghee, continue to cook. In 5 to 10 more minutes, the milk solids that were not skimmed off will settle to the bottom of the pan and start to brown. Cook for 4 to 5 more minutes to enhance the richness of the flavour.

3. Remove from the heat and let the ghee cool for a few minutes. Pour it through cheesecloth or a fine-mesh strainer into a mason jar to strain out any remaining milk proteins.

4. After straining the finished ghee into the mason jar, stir in the turmeric. It will likely settle to the bottom right away. Stir every hour for a few hours until the ghee has turned solid. When the ghee is completely cool, seal with a lid. Store in the fridge for up to 6 months.

Italian-Seasoned Ghee
Gluten-free • Grain-free • Nut-free • Vegetarian

1 pound (450 g) unsalted butter, cubed
1 teaspoon (5 mL) Italian seasoning

1. Melt the butter in a medium pot, preferably with a heavy bottom so it doesn't easily burn, over medium heat. Once the butter melts, it will start to bubble and the milk proteins will begin to separate from the fat and float to the surface. Using a spoon, skim off these milk proteins. Reduce the heat to medium-low and continue cooking until the ghee is clear and you've skimmed off all the protein, 15 to 20 minutes.

2. Once it's clear, you have clarified butter, but to make ghee, continue to cook. In 5 to 10 more minutes, the milk solids that were not skimmed off will settle to the bottom of the pan and start to brown. Cook for 4 to 5 more minutes to enhance the richness of the flavour.

3. Remove from the heat and let the ghee cool for a few minutes. Pour it through cheesecloth or a fine-mesh strainer into a mason jar to strain out any remaining milk proteins.

4. After straining the finished ghee into the mason jar, stir in the Italian seasoning. It will likely settle to the bottom right away. Stir every hour for a few hours until the ghee has turned solid. When the ghee is completely cool, seal with a lid. Store in the fridge for up to 6 months.

Toast Six Ways

Each variation serves 1

We eat a lot of toast in my family. It's so versatile—it can be sweet, savoury, salty, whatever your heart desires. Toast need not be boring. Toast to me is comforting, and can be either easy or as complicated and fancy as you want it to be. My go-to is topped with almond butter and sliced apple or banana.

The quality of the bread is what separates great toast from mediocre. We love sourdough bread in our home—it's serious business. The fermentation of the dough lowers the gluten content and makes it far more digestible. My favourite sourdough is buckwheat sourdough. We always have a variety of breads in our freezer, and on our kitchen counter we always have a loaf of sourdough from our local bakery.

Ginger Guacamole Radish Toast

Dairy-free • Kid-friendly • Nut-free • Vegan

1 slice of your favourite sourdough bread, toasted
¼ cup (60 mL) Ginger Sesame Guacamole (page 73)
1 to 2 radishes, thinly sliced
Handful of pea sprouts
Sea salt

1. Spread the Ginger Sesame Guacamole on the toast and top with radish slices, pea sprouts and sea salt to taste.

Ricotta Raspberry Toast

Kid-friendly • Nut-free • Vegetarian

1 slice of your favourite sourdough bread, toasted
3 to 4 tablespoons (45 to 60 mL) ricotta cheese
5 fresh raspberries
Drizzle of pure liquid honey
¼ teaspoon (1 mL) chopped fresh mint

1. Spread the ricotta on the toast and top with raspberries, honey and mint.

Beet Cucumber Toast

Kid-friendly • Nut-free • Vegetarian

1 slice of your favourite sourdough bread, toasted
¼ cup (60 mL) Roasted Beet and Garlic Dip (page 77)
4 or 5 slices of English cucumber
Sprinkle of crumbled goat cheese
Pinch of dried rosemary
Sea salt and pepper

1. Spread the Roasted Beet and Garlic Dip on the toast and top with cucumber, goat cheese, dried rosemary, and sea salt and pepper to taste.

recipe continues

Almond Butter Apple Toast
Dairy-free • Kid-friendly • Vegan

1 slice of your favourite sourdough bread, toasted
2 tablespoons (30 mL) natural almond butter
3 or 4 apple slices (Royal Gala, McIntosh or Granny Smith)
Pinch of cinnamon
½ teaspoon (2 mL) hemp seeds

1. Spread the almond butter on the toast and top with apple slices, cinnamon and hemp seeds.

Sunflower Butter Banana Toast
Dairy-free • Kid-friendly • Nut-free • Vegan

1 slice of your favourite sourdough bread, toasted
2 tablespoons (30 mL) natural sunflower butter
4 slices of ripe banana
¼ teaspoon (1 mL) raw cacao nibs or dairy-free chocolate chips
Pinch of cinnamon

1. Spread the sunflower butter on the toast and top with banana slices, cacao nibs and cinnamon.

Eggy Toast
Dairy-free • Kid-friendly • Vegetarian

1 egg
1 tablespoon (15 mL) unsweetened almond milk or cashew milk
½ teaspoon (2 mL) coconut oil
½ ripe avocado, pitted, peeled and thinly sliced
1 slice of your favourite sourdough bread, toasted
4 grape tomatoes, cut in half
Pinch of garlic powder
Dash of hot sauce
Sea salt and pepper

1. In a small bowl, whisk together the egg and almond milk.

2. Heat the coconut oil in a small frying pan over medium heat. Pour the egg mixture into the pan and let cook, without stirring, for about 30 seconds. Stir with a spoon for 3 to 4 minutes, until no visible liquid egg remains but the egg is not dry, either.

3. Arrange the avocado slices on the toast and top with the scrambled egg, tomatoes, garlic powder, hot sauce, and sea salt and pepper to taste.

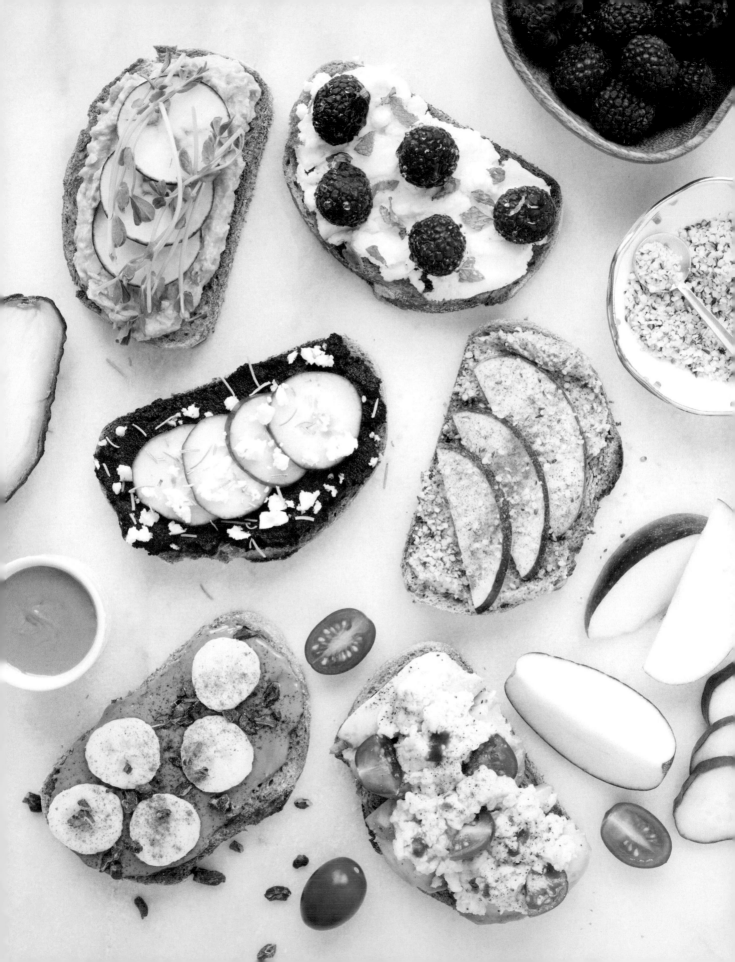

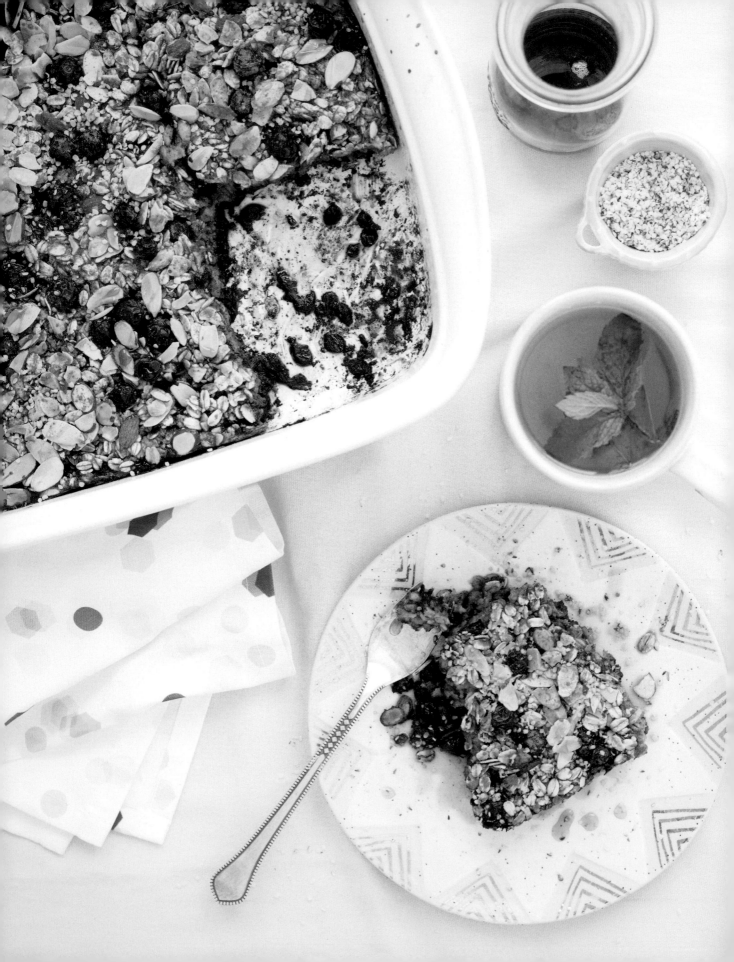

Baked Blueberry Almond Hemp Oatmeal

Dairy-free • Kid-friendly • Vegetarian

Serves 6 to 8

My good friend Carol, who also happens to be the food stylist for my cookbooks and someone I've worked with for nearly a decade, has been talking about her blueberry bake for years. In fact, we discussed putting her recipe in my first cookbook, *Joyous Health*. I finally twisted Carol's arm and she graciously shared her recipe with me. Lucky for us all, because it's absolutely delicious and everything you'd ever want comfort food to be.

This decadent baked oatmeal is a lovely alternative to pancakes or waffles for Sunday brunch, or put some aside so you can enjoy it throughout the week—it warms up nicely in the oven. If you use frozen blueberries, make sure you let them thaw and drain before using, or the blueberry bake may be too mushy. This is definitely on the sweeter side, so you may not even need to serve with maple syrup. This recipe works as a dessert too, with a nice dollop of vanilla coconut milk ice cream on top.

3 cups (750 mL) fresh or drained thawed frozen blueberries, divided

3 cups (750 mL) oat flakes or old-fashioned rolled oats

¼ cup (60 mL) coconut sugar

1 tablespoon (15 mL) cinnamon

½ teaspoon (2 mL) sea salt

2 eggs

2 cups (500 mL) unsweetened almond milk or your favourite nut milk

⅓ cup (75 mL) real maple syrup, more for serving

1 tablespoon (15 mL) pure vanilla extract

⅔ cup (150 mL) slivered raw almonds

¼ cup (60 mL) hemp seeds

1. Preheat the oven to 350°F (180°C). Grease the bottom and sides of a 13- × 9-inch (3.5 L) baking dish with coconut oil.

2. Spread 2½ cups (625 mL) of the blueberries in the baking dish.

3. In a medium bowl, stir together the oats, coconut sugar, cinnamon and sea salt.

4. In a small bowl, whisk the eggs, then whisk in the almond milk, maple syrup and vanilla.

5. Sprinkle the oat mixture evenly over the blueberries. Then pour the almond milk mixture over the oat mixture. Gently shake the dish to make sure the milk mixture evenly covers the oats. Scatter the remaining ½ cup (125 mL) blueberries and the slivered almonds evenly over the top. Bake until golden brown, 30 to 45 minutes.

6. Sprinkle with hemp seeds just before serving. Serve warm drizzled with maple syrup.

7. Store covered in the fridge for up to 5 days. Enjoy leftovers chilled or reheat in the oven at 350°F (180°C) for 10 minutes.

Beet Smoothie Bowl

Dairy-free • Gluten-free • Kid-friendly • Vegetarian

Serves 2

The beautiful colour of this smoothie is proof of its health benefits. The rich red comes from phytonutrients called betalains that provide antioxidant, anti-inflammatory and detoxification support. It doesn't stop there, because this recipe includes cauliflower, which has incredible anti-cancer nutrients. If you're wondering how a smoothie bowl can possibly taste good with cauliflower in it, don't worry: the other ingredients mask its flavour. For convenience, most grocery stores sell pre-cooked frozen cauliflower, so you don't have to prep and cook a head of cauliflower just for this smoothie. If you don't have cauliflower on hand, zucchini is a great swap and doesn't need to be cooked first.

The chocolate protein powder, honey and coconut butter are essential for flavour. If you don't have chocolate protein powder, just add 2 to 3 tablespoons (30 to 45 mL) of raw cacao powder, depending how chocolaty you like your smoothie. If you have a few extra minutes, use cookie cutters in different shapes and sizes to make cut-outs from slices of fruit, such as apple or kiwi, to decorate the smoothie bowls.

2 small raw red beets (unpeeled if organic), chopped

2 cups (500 mL) fresh or thawed frozen strawberries

1 cup (250 mL) cooked cauliflower florets

½ cup (125 mL) unsweetened plain full-fat coconut yogurt

¼ cup (60 mL) plant-based chocolate protein powder

2 tablespoons (30 mL) raw liquid honey

2 tablespoons (30 mL) coconut butter

1 cup (250 mL) unsweetened nut milk of your choice

Filtered water, just enough for desired consistency

Fruit cut-outs, for garnish (optional)

1. Place all the ingredients, except the water, in a high-speed blender. Blend for 30 to 60 seconds, until smooth, adding the water only as needed.

2. Divide between 2 bowls and top with fruit cut-outs, if using. If you have leftovers, store in an airtight container in the fridge for up to 1 day or in the freezer for up to 2 weeks.

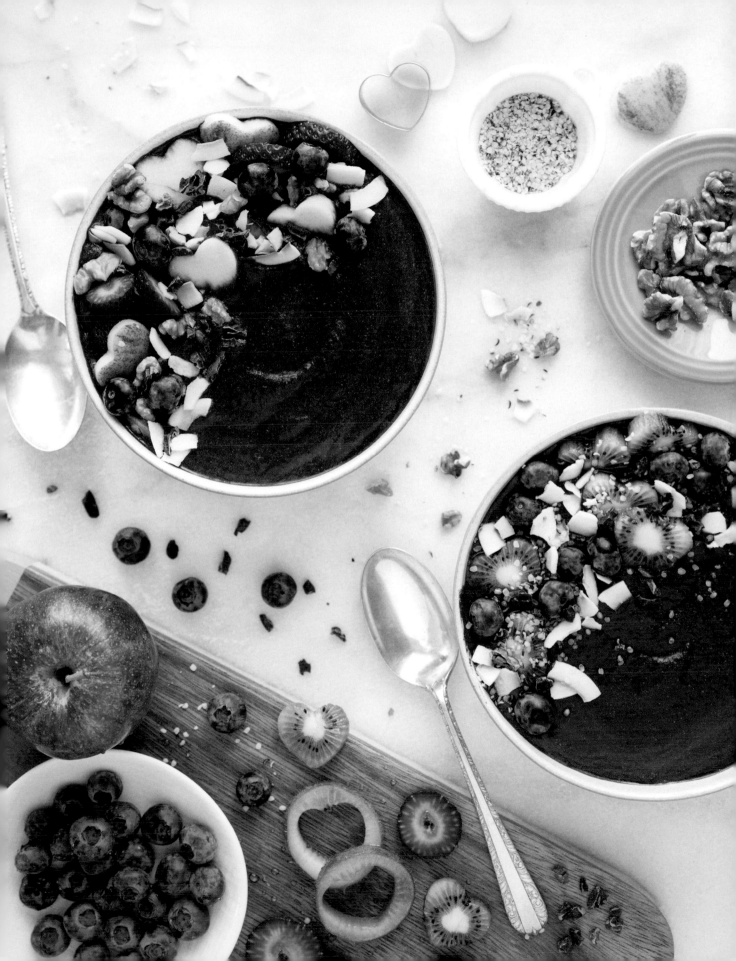

Maca Chocolate Almond Butter Smoothie

Dairy-free • Gluten-free • Kid-friendly • Vegan

Serves 2

Maca, chocolate and almond butter—combinations don't get any better than that. This is one of those smoothies that works 365 days a year. I love making it in the hot, humid days of summer to cool off, and on frigid winter mornings, this smoothie offers comfort because it's rich and fulfilling. Even though this is intended as a breakfast smoothie, it could be a snack if you halved it or a dessert smoothie for a boost of energy and vitality!

The creaminess of this smoothie is thanks to the avocado. Avocados are my secret weapon for the perfect smoothie texture every single time. The good monounsaturated fats in them are anti-inflammatory and skin-loving in every way. If you don't have chocolate-flavoured protein powder on hand, plain will do fine, but taste test and add more cacao powder if need be. Almond milk is ideal in this smoothie, as it complements all the flavours, but any nut milk or rice milk will do. If you want to take the flavour to a whole new delicious level, then I recommend adding espresso for a nice hit of caffeine—my husband Walker's favourite way to enjoy this smoothie. If serving kids, I suggest skipping the espresso!

1 ripe avocado, pitted, peeled and roughly chopped

1 ripe banana, roughly chopped

3 tablespoons (45 mL) raw cacao powder

3 tablespoons (45 mL) natural almond butter

2 heaping tablespoons (36 mL) plant-based chocolate protein powder

2 tablespoons (30 mL) real maple syrup

2 teaspoons (10 mL) maca root powder

1 cup (250 mL) unsweetened nut milk

2 shots (1 ounce/30 mL each) espresso (optional)

Filtered water, just enough for desired consistency

1. Place all the ingredients, except the water, in a high-speed blender. Blend for 30 to 60 seconds, until smooth, adding the water only as needed.

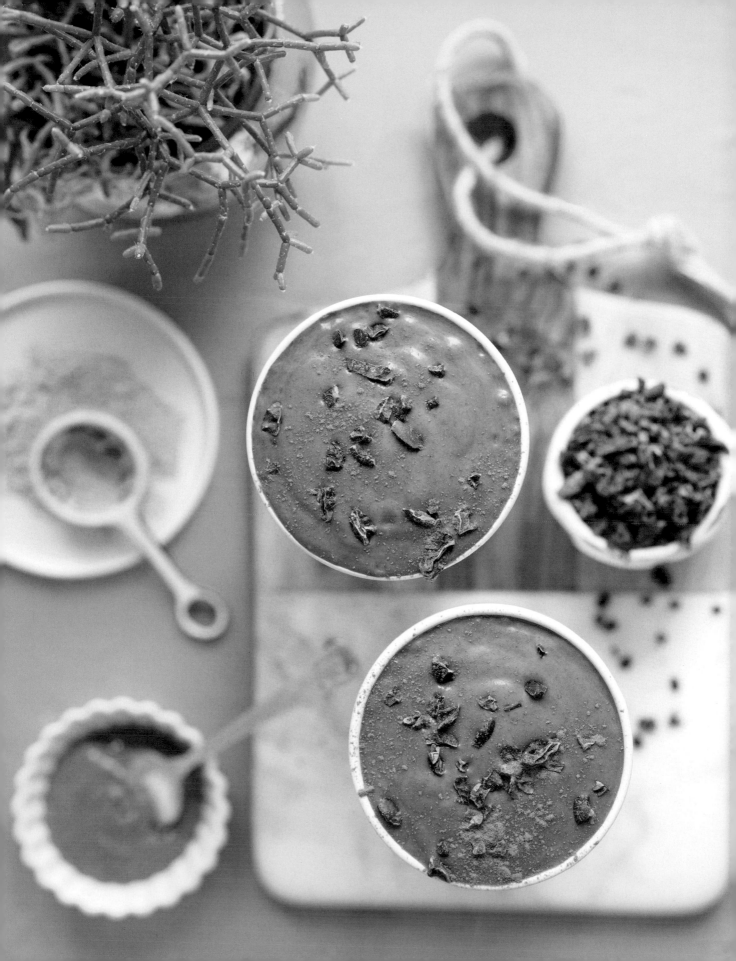

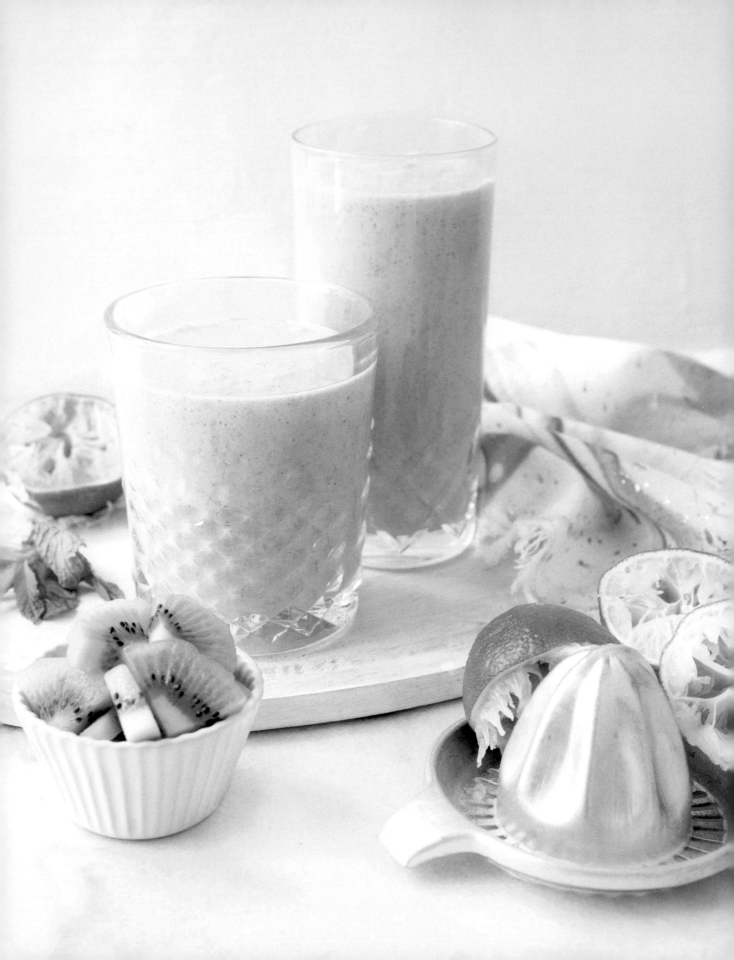

Green Mojito Smoothie
Dairy-free • Gluten-free • Grain-free • Kid-friendly • Nut-free • Vegan

Serves 2

Smoothies have been my go-to on weekday mornings ever since I was pregnant with Vienna. I realized I couldn't stomach much in the morning but I still wanted something healthy. These days I often make a smoothie to share with my hubs, Walker, and Vienna a few mornings a week, even in winter.

Smoothies are such an easy way to pack a truckload of nutrients into one delicious cup. You get tons of fibre to fill you up, antioxidants like vitamin C, B vitamins for energy, good fat to fill your belly and loads of flavour. This creamy smoothie reminds me of a mojito because of the mint. It's super refreshing and nourishing. When our mornings are busy, I enjoy this smoothie with one of my Applesauce Spice Breakfast Muffins (page 18) and I'm satisfied until lunch.

1 ripe avocado, pitted, peeled and
   roughly chopped
3 kiwis, peeled and roughly chopped
2 cups (500 mL) frozen pineapple chunks
1 cup (250 mL) loosely packed fresh
   baby spinach or kale
¼ cup (60 mL) fresh mint leaves
1 can (14 ounces/398 mL) full-fat
   coconut milk
Juice of 3 limes
1 cup (250 mL) ice
Filtered water, just enough for desired
   consistency

1. Place all the ingredients, except the water, in a high-speed blender. Blend for 30 to 60 seconds, until smooth, adding the water only as needed.

Lemon Blueberry Cashew Smoothie
Kid-friendly • Vegetarian

Serves 2

I love smoothies because you can slurp your way to sustained energy and great digestion when you don't have time for anything else. Few days go by that I don't have a smoothie. These days I don't make my smoothies as "green" as I used to because I almost always share them with my daughter. I can easily down super-green smoothies, but for Vienna they just aren't as palatable as this one.

I make most smoothies with whatever I have handy. I don't shop specifically for my smoothies, but there are always berries in my fridge or freezer and I always have some nuts or seeds on hand. I also always make sure I have some kind of nut milk. I love the creaminess of cashew milk, and it's fairly easy to find at large grocery stores nowadays, but if you can't find any, just use almond milk or whatever you can get your hands on.

1½ cups (375 mL) fresh or thawed frozen blueberries

1 cup (250 mL) unsweetened plain full-fat coconut yogurt or sheep's milk yogurt

½ cup (125 mL) oat flakes

½ cup (125 mL) raw cashews

5 Medjool dates, pitted

Zest and juice of 1 lemon

1 cup (250 mL) unsweetened cashew milk or other nut milk

Filtered water, just enough for desired consistency

1. Place all the ingredients, except the water, in a high-speed blender. Blend for 30 to 60 seconds, until smooth, adding the water only as needed.

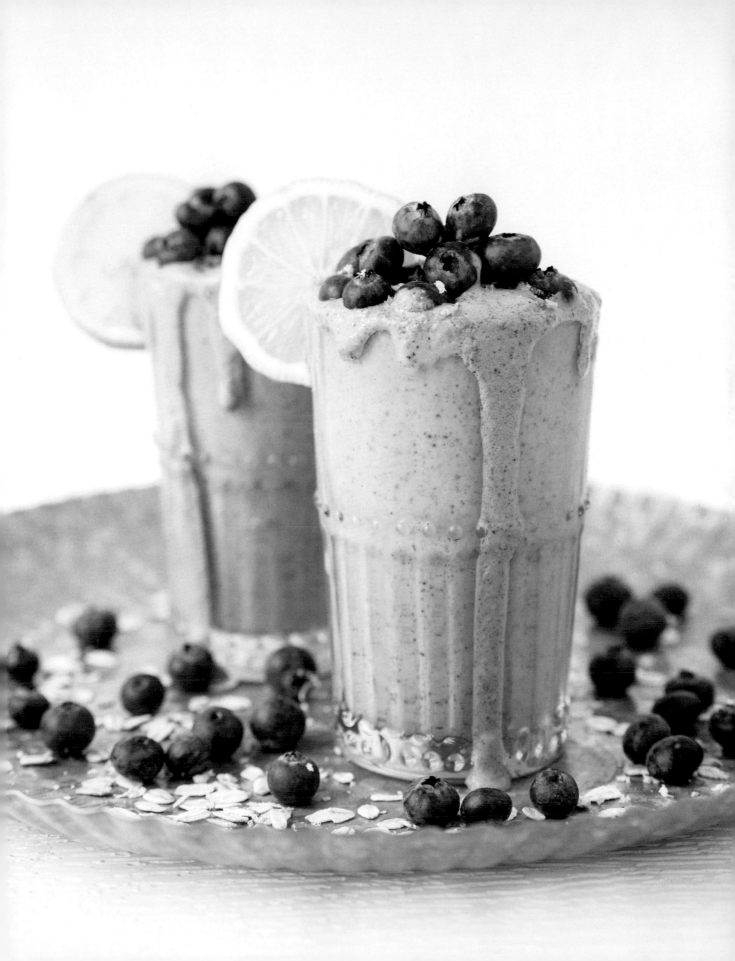

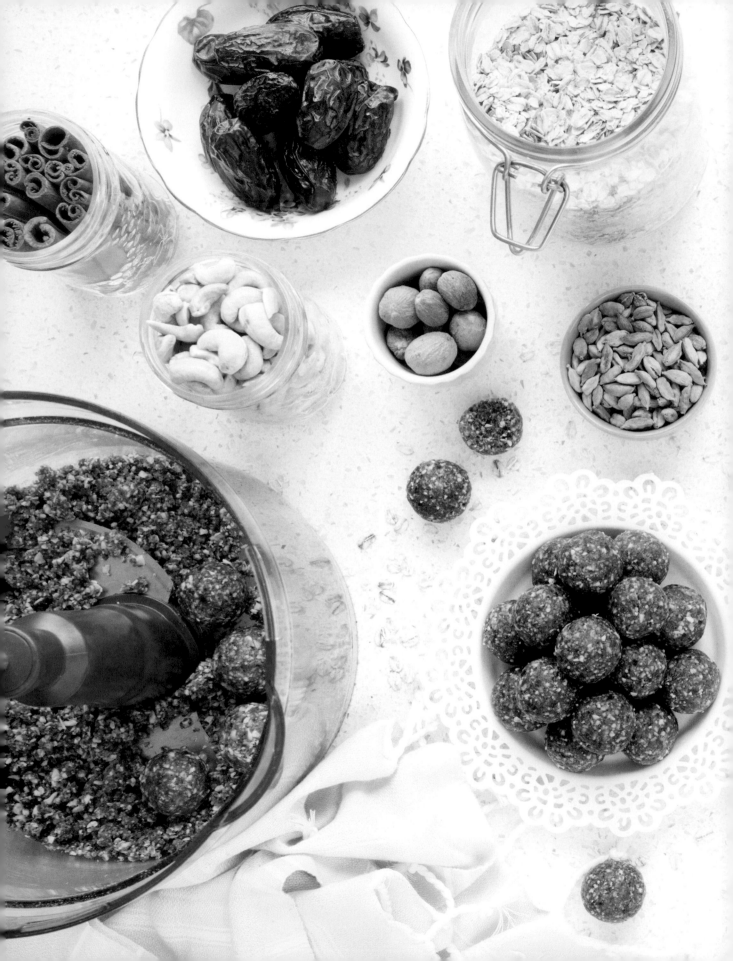

Drinks and Snacks

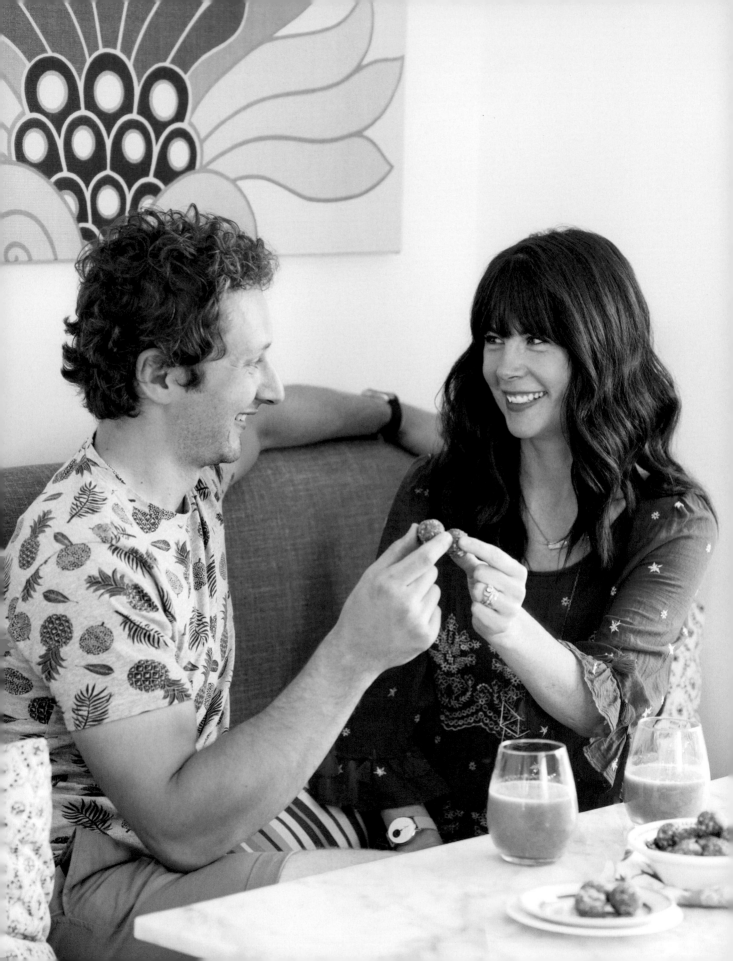

DRINKS AND SNACKS

These recipes are for those times between meals when you are hungry but just want a little something to tide you over till lunch or dinner. They are also perfect after-school snacks for kids. Our daughter, Vienna, is always ravenous when she gets home from school, so I make sure I have some nourishing snacks ready to go to put something in her belly but still leave room for dinner. I love feeling hungry before a meal, so I make sure I don't ruin my appetite by eating heavy snacks. This is why I love wellness drinks like my Turmeric Ginger Latte (page 69) and the refreshing Green Juice Spritzer (page 62), or a light snack such as Cauliflower Hummus (page 78) with crunchy raw veggies.

Craving a sugary snack or caffeinated beverage during those in-between times is typically a sign that your blood sugar has dipped. Your body is looking for a quick boost of energy! The problem is that sugary snacks and caffeinated drinks don't provide long-lasting energy. They may actually have the opposite effect and drain you of energy and vitality. Who needs that when you've got things to do and people to see. But you can satisfy your sweet tooth *and* have a nourishing snack! Something like a couple of Oat, Spice and Everything Nice Balls (page 86) will balance blood sugar, keep away sugar cravings and keep you feeling joyous until your next main meal.

Green Juice Spritzer

Dairy-free • Gluten-free • Grain-free • Nut-free • Vegan

Serves 2

Most green juices are a morning ritual for me—a great way to start the day by cleansing, nourishing and detoxing my body. However, when I need to hit the reset button in the middle of the day, I love adding sparkling water to a green juice to turn it into a spritzer that's even more refreshing and thirst-quenching. This spritzer is also a wonderful option when you're entertaining because it's always a hit with those who don't drink alcohol but still want something bubbly and refreshing.

This is a green juice I come back to again and again. The combination of lime, basil and cucumber is truly delightful! I love making it when I've got basil growing and I need to use up my leafy greens before they go limp in my fridge. If you do not have a juice extractor, you can cut the apple and cucumber into chunks and blend everything in a high-speed blender, then strain through a nut bag or fine-mesh strainer.

1 apple (Granny Smith, Royal Gala or McIntosh)

1 field cucumber

2 limes

2 cups (500 mL) tightly packed baby spinach or kale

¼ cup (60 mL) loosely packed fresh basil leaves

1 to 2 cups (250 to 500 mL) sparkling water

1. Cut the apple, cucumber and limes into small chunks that will fit in the mouth of your juice extractor. Remove the seeds from the apple. Run all the ingredients, except the sparkling water, through the juice extractor. Divide between 2 glasses and top up with sparkling water.

2. Refrigerate any leftover spritzer but drink within 6 hours for optimal freshness.

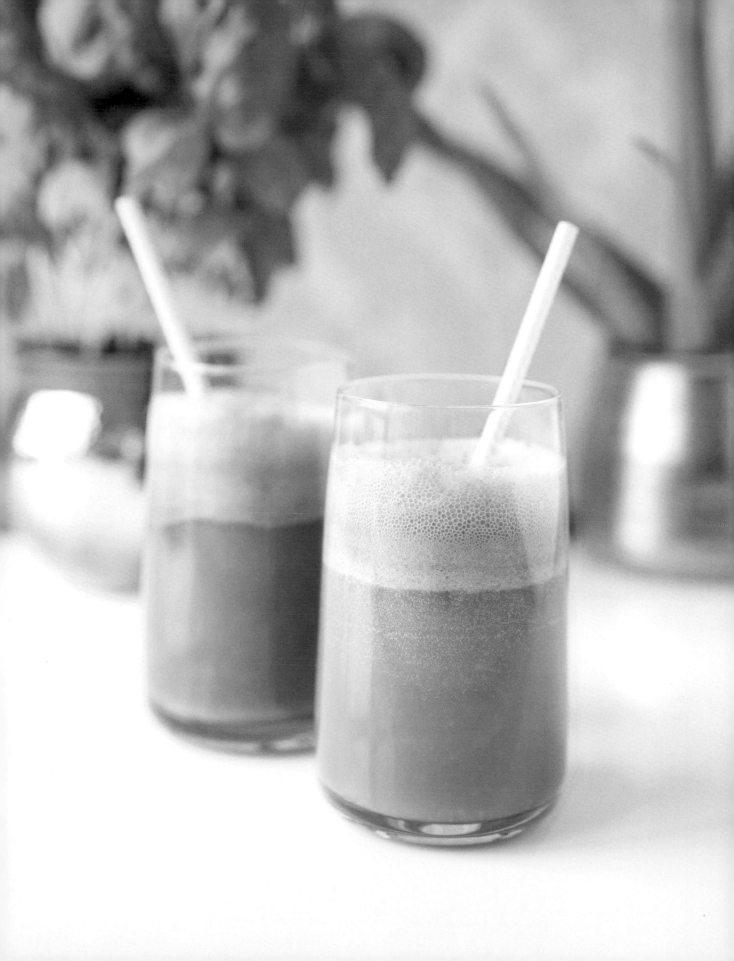

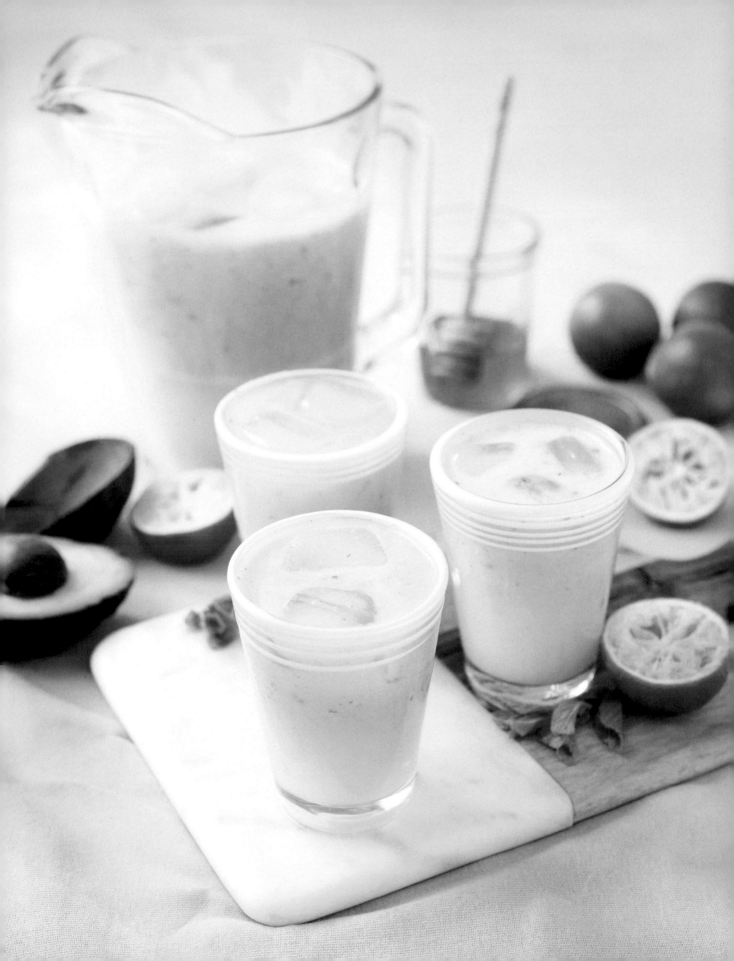

Avocado Lime Refresher

Dairy-free • Gluten-free • Grain-free • Kid-friendly • Nut-free • Vegetarian

Serves 8 to 10

I travelled to Mexico for a yoga retreat several years ago, but I still remember the smell and taste of this drink that greeted me when I arrived at the resort. Little did I know it would also greet me after every single yoga class. It was refreshing, slightly sweet and super hydrating. I was staying in a grass hut with a mosquito net for sleeping. It was steamy, humid and hot, all day and all night, so this Avocado Lime Refresher was the perfect thing to revive my body after our morning yoga sessions. I love making this for summer barbecues when it's hot and steamy outside. It's always a hit at family gatherings instead of sugar-filled drinks like lemonade and punch.

½ ripe avocado, pitted, peeled and
    roughly chopped
Juice of 3 limes
6 cups (1.5 L) coconut water
2 tablespoons (30 mL) pure liquid honey,
    more as needed
2 tablespoons (30 mL) fresh mint leaves
1 cup (250 mL) ice

1. Place all the ingredients, except the ice, in a high-speed blender. Blend for 30 to 60 seconds, until smooth. Taste and add up to 1 tablespoon (15 mL) more honey, if needed, for desired sweetness and blend for 30 more seconds. Chill for 2 hours.

2. Before serving, pour into a big jug, add the ice and give it a stir.

Honey Lemon Cayenne Elixir

Dairy-free • Gluten-free • Grain-free • Nut-free • Vegetarian

Makes about 1 cup (250 mL), 18 to 20 servings

This elixir has incredible health benefits for detoxification and the immune system (wonderful to soothe a sore throat), but sometimes I add a tablespoon or two to hot water just to warm me up on a cold day. And occasionally I will have it straight up on a spoon. Be forewarned, the ginger and cayenne make it pretty fiery! I use a small amount of cayenne, but often add more on those days I need an extra boost for my metabolism.

When adding the ingredients to your mason jar, you may not use the full amount of honey—make sure to leave enough room for the ingredients to move around when you shake the jar.

2 to 3 lemons, cut into chunks
2-inch (5 cm) piece of fresh turmeric,
　peeled and sliced lengthwise
　(or 1 teaspoon/5 mL ground turmeric)
2 tablespoons (30 mL) grated fresh ginger
1 cup (250 mL) pure liquid honey
⅛ teaspoon (0.5 mL) cayenne pepper

1. Place the lemons, turmeric and ginger in a 2-cup (500 mL) wide-mouth mason jar. Pour the honey over top, leaving about ¾ inch (2 cm) space from the top. Sprinkle in the cayenne. Tighten the lid and give the jar a good shake.

2. Pour 1 to 2 tablespoons (15 to 30 mL) into a glass of hot filtered water or enjoy as a shot with 2 ounces (60 mL) of warm filtered water. Store in the fridge for up to 2 weeks or in the freezer for up to 3 months.

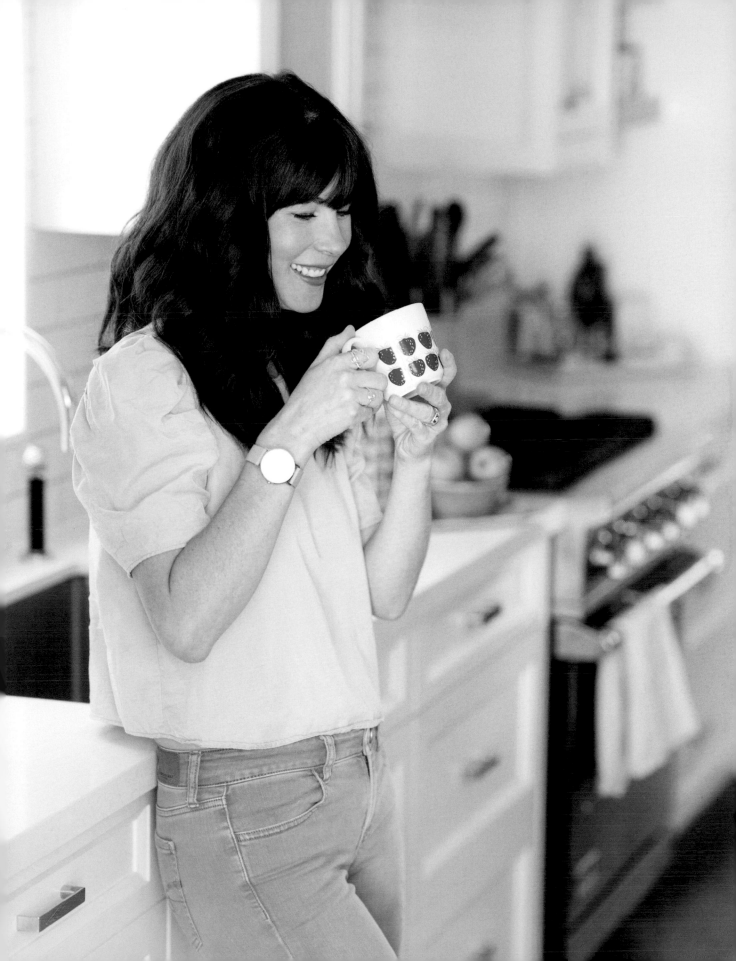

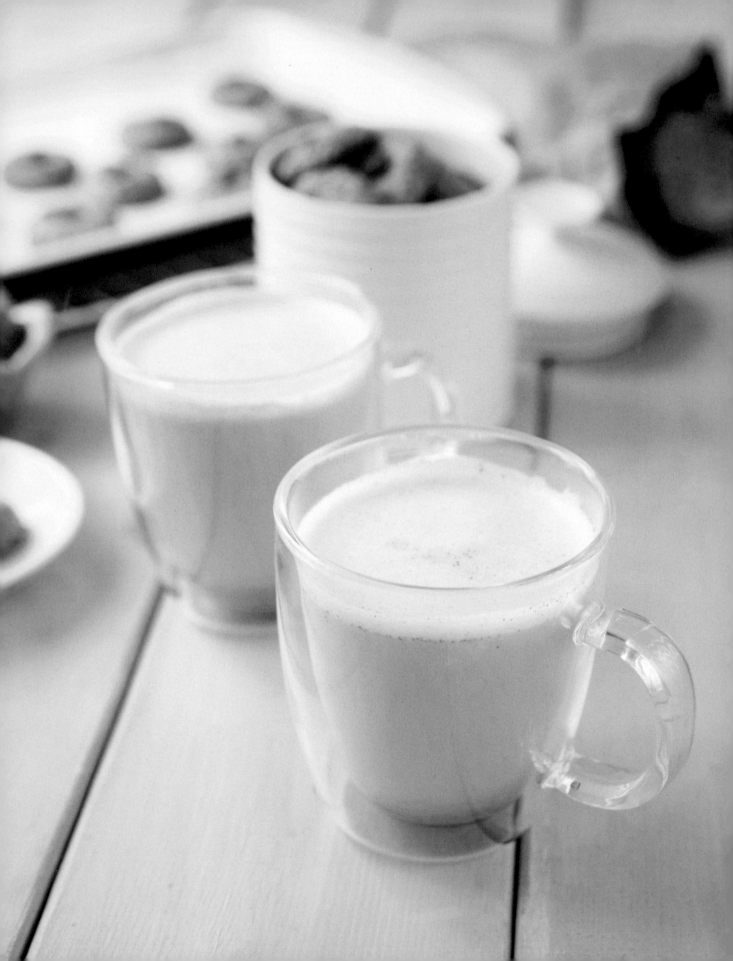

Turmeric Ginger Latte

Dairy-free • Gluten-free • Grain-free • Nut-free • Vegan

Serves 2

This is my favourite drink of all time. In the summer I enjoy it with ice and in the winter it warms me up on a cold day. Turmeric is the star of this latte—one of my favourite superfoods and one of the most researched foods in modern science. Turmeric is an incredibly detoxifying, anti-inflammatory and antioxidant-rich food. Many people shy away from turmeric, thinking it will make everything taste like curry. But turmeric all on its own is both sweet and savoury. So no, this latte doesn't taste like curry. It tastes like heaven!

Coconut butter gives this drink a wonderful natural sweetness and creaminess. It's a worthy investment, but if you don't have any on hand, you can easily make up for the lack of sweetness with a touch of maple syrup. For the creaminess, you could swap out half the hot water for coconut milk instead.

3 heaping tablespoons (54 mL) coconut butter

1 tablespoon (15 mL) real maple syrup (optional)

2 teaspoons (10 mL) ground turmeric (or 4 teaspoons/20 mL grated peeled fresh turmeric)

1 teaspoon (5 mL) grated fresh ginger

½ teaspoon (2 mL) cinnamon

2 cups (500 mL) hot filtered water

1. Place all the ingredients in a high-speed blender. Depending on how hot your water is, you may need to let the steam dissipate before you put the lid on your blender. Blend for 30 to 60 seconds, until smooth. Some sediment might settle at the bottom of your cup. If you wish to avoid this, strain the drink through a fine-mesh strainer when pouring from the blender.

Nighty Night Tea
Dairy-free • Gluten-free • Grain-free • Nut-free • Vegan

Makes enough for 24 cups of tea

I've been a tea drinker for as long as I can remember. In the cooler months I drink tea in both the morning and the evening, but in the summer I typically have tea only in the evening. Even on hot summer nights, I still brew a cup of tea before bed. It's a ritual I love, and it helps prepare my body for a restful sleep. I absolutely love this tea, as the passionflower, chamomile and hops all have relaxing and calming medicinal properties. Passionflower helps induce sleep and it has long been used to ease nervousness, anxiety and agitation. Chamomile has been used in traditional medicine for those who suffer from sleep apnea, restless sleep or mild anxiety, and its phenolic compounds help to strengthen the immune system. Most people know of hops in relation to beer, but they are a mild natural sedative—a perfect ingredient for relaxation.

I buy the dried herbs from my local herbal dispensary and store the mix in a mason jar for optimal freshness. Once the tea is brewed, I add some honey or a few drops of organic liquid stevia for a touch of sweetness.

½ cup (125 mL) dried passionflower
½ cup (125 mL) dried chamomile flowers
½ cup (125 mL) dried hops flowers

1. Stir together all the ingredients. Store in a mason jar out of direct light and away from heat for up to 3 months.

2. To brew a cup of tea, add 1 tablespoon (15 mL) tea mixture to 1 cup (250 mL) boiling water. Let steep for 4 to 5 minutes.

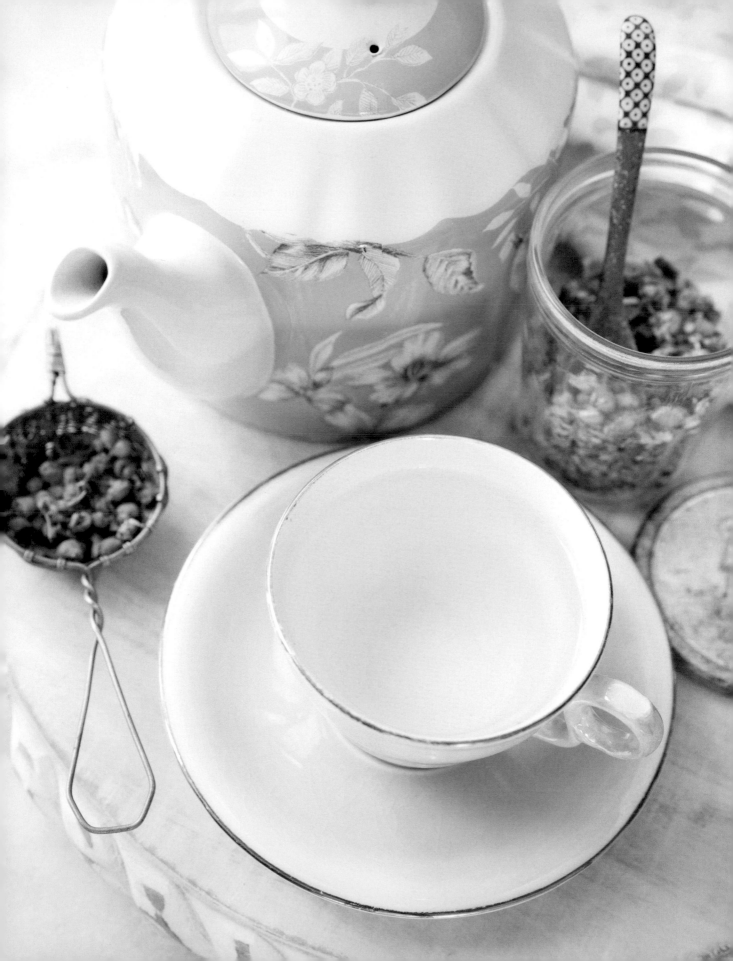

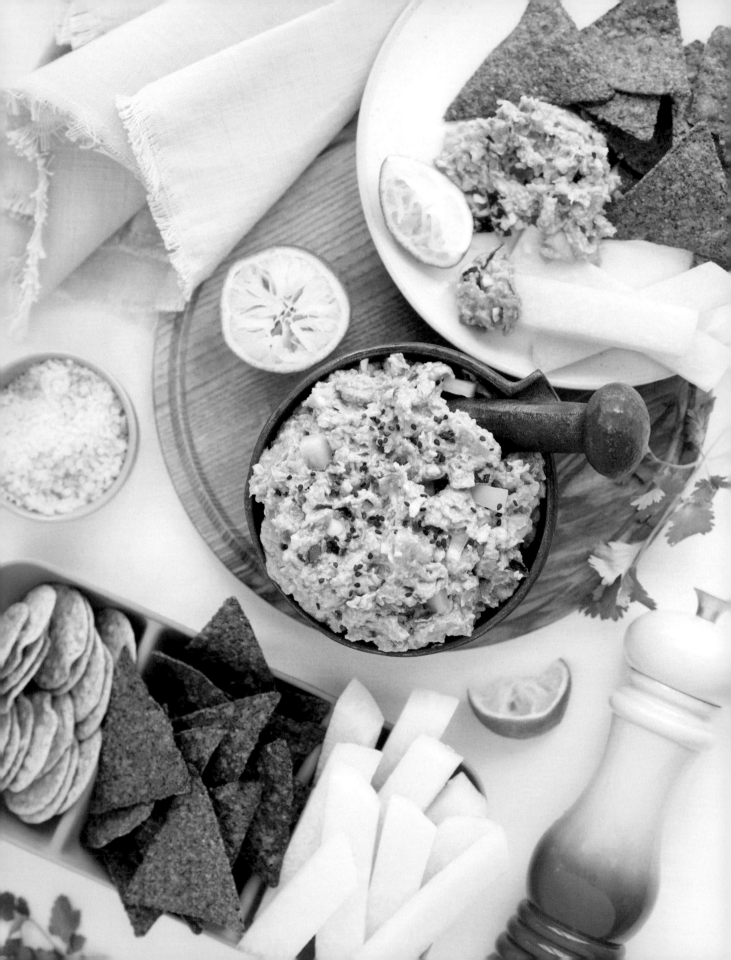

Ginger Sesame Guacamole

Dairy-free • Gluten-free • Grain-free • Kid-friendly • Nut-free • Vegan

Serves 4

Every Christmas we visit my in-laws in south Florida, and we always make time for lunch at a restaurant called the Avocado Grill. From salads to tacos, pretty much every item on the menu contains avocado. And yes, they have guacamole. After all, they really couldn't be called the Avocado Grill if they didn't have guacamole!

This ginger guacamole was inspired by one I had at the restaurant. This might not be a combination you would think would work, but it really does! The ginger totally brightens up the flavour and makes for a memorable guac. Winter, spring, summer or fall, I'm always in the mood for ginger guac. It's a crowd-pleaser kid-friendly and nutritionist-approved thanks to all those good fats and fibre. I love to serve it with sliced jicama and corn chips.

4 ripe avocados, pitted and peeled
1 sweet yellow or orange pepper, finely chopped
¼ red onion, finely chopped
1 to 2 cloves garlic, finely chopped
¼ cup (60 mL) chopped fresh cilantro
1 tablespoon (15 mL) grated fresh ginger
Juice of 2 limes
1 tablespoon (15 mL) white or black sesame seeds

1. In a large bowl, mash the avocados with a fork. Add the yellow pepper, red onion, garlic, cilantro, ginger and lime juice. Stir until mixed. Transfer to a serving bowl and sprinkle with sesame seeds before serving.

Walker's Navy Bean Spread

Dairy-free • Kid-friendly • Nut-free • Vegan

Serves 6

This is a joyous family favourite! When my hubs, Walker, and I have a date night, we often go to a nearby Italian restaurant, where we always order the tuna navy bean crostini as an appetizer to share. Walker decided to re-create it one afternoon without the tuna (because we didn't have any), and it has since become a homemade favourite. We make it often, either when entertaining or on lazy weekend afternoons when we're feeling peckish by mid-afternoon but don't want to eat too much and spoil our dinner. It's fresh, flavourful and full of plant-based protein and fibre. Sometimes we add chopped celery for crunch. You can enjoy it on crackers or—my preference—sourdough bread toasted in the oven with some extra-virgin olive oil and dried rosemary.

I like to use a fork or a potato masher to crush the beans because I like some of them to remain intact. Alternatively, a food processor will provide a nice smooth texture like hummus. You may just need to add a little more olive oil or a splash of water for a thinner consistency. Either way, it's delicious!

2 cans (15 ounces/425 mL each) navy beans, drained and rinsed

2 cloves garlic, minced

Juice of 2 lemons

4 tablespoons (60 mL) extra-virgin olive oil, divided

½ teaspoon (2 mL) sea salt, divided

½ cup (125 mL) loosely packed chopped fresh flat-leaf parsley

¼ cup (60 mL) chopped green onions (white and light green parts only)

1 sourdough baguette, sliced

½ teaspoon (2 mL) dried rosemary

1. Preheat the oven to 375°F (190°C). Line a baking sheet with parchment paper.

2. In a large bowl, combine the navy beans, garlic, lemon juice, 2 tablespoons (30 mL) of the olive oil and ¼ teaspoon (1 mL) of the sea salt. Mash together with a fork or a potato masher.

3. Add the parsley and green onions and stir together.

4. Arrange the sliced baguette evenly on the prepared baking sheet. Drizzle with the remaining 2 tablespoons (30 mL) olive oil and sprinkle with the rosemary and remaining ¼ teaspoon (1 mL) sea salt. Toast until golden and crunchy, 10 to 12 minutes.

5. Spread the desired amount of dip on each piece of toasted baguette and serve right away.

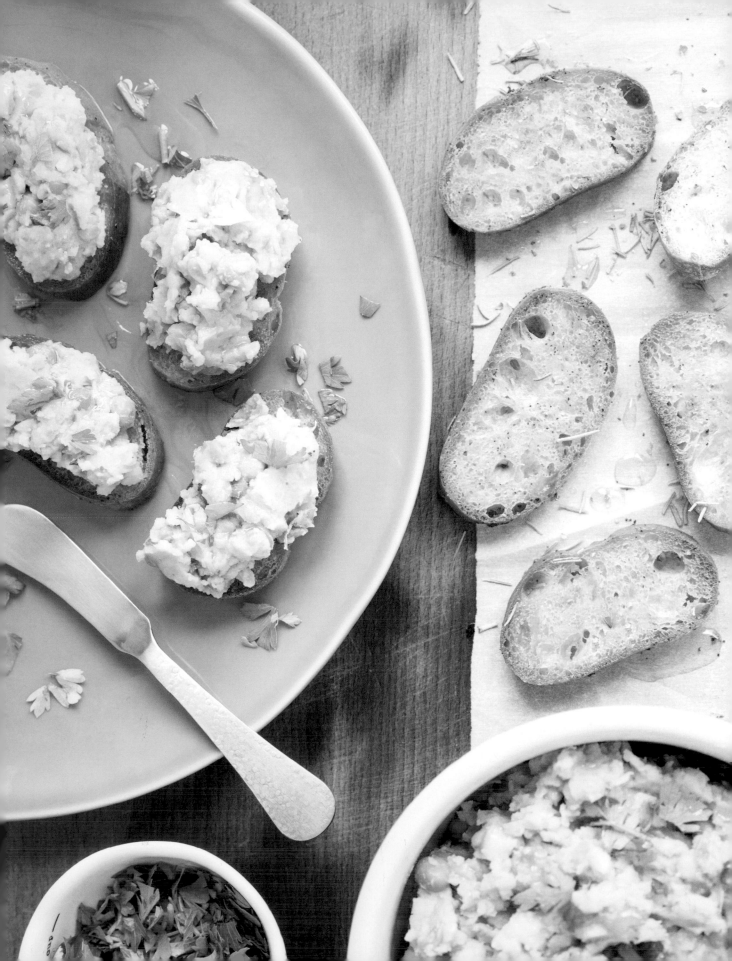

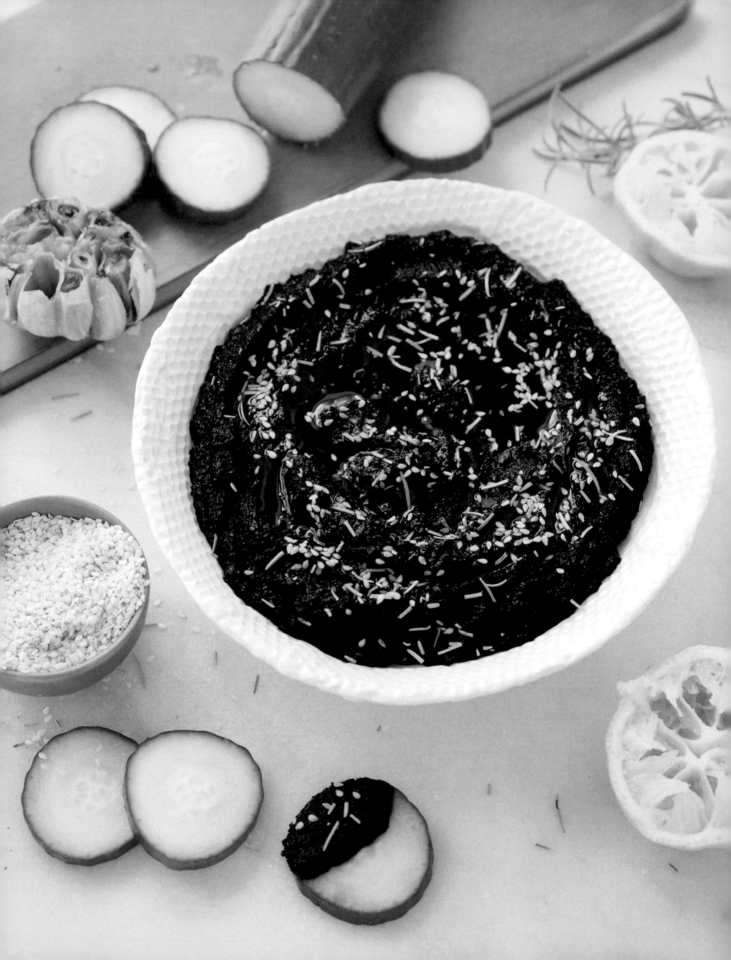

Roasted Beet and Garlic Dip

Dairy-free • Gluten-free • Grain-free • Kid-friendly • Nut-free • Vegan

Makes 2 to 3 cups (500 to 750 mL)

I adore roasted beets so I just assume everyone else loves beets, but that's not always the case. If you're one of those people who find their earthy taste a bit much, I promise I can change your mind with this super-creamy and incredibly flavourful dip. The roasted garlic adds a wonderful flavour that's not overpowering, but if you don't have time to roast it, you can use fresh garlic instead—but you will only need one to two cloves of fresh garlic, not the whole bulb! From a health perspective beets are absolute superstars. They contain a plethora of phytonutrients that aid your liver in detoxification. They are also blood-building and energizing. And kids love this dip, so it's a surefire winner for the whole family.

If you're entertaining, serve this dip along with my Cauliflower Hummus (page 78) and you'll have two winners at your party! I like to serve the dips with either cucumber slices or brown rice crackers.

5 medium red beets (unpeeled if organic), roughly chopped

1 whole garlic bulb

½ teaspoon (2 mL) + ¼ cup (60 mL) extra-virgin olive oil, divided, more for serving

¼ cup (60 mL) tahini

1 teaspoon (5 mL) dried rosemary

½ teaspoon (2 mL) sea salt

1 tablespoon (15 mL) sesame seeds, for garnish

1. Preheat the oven to 350°F (180°C).

2. Place the chopped beets in a large baking dish and add enough water to come ¼ inch (5 mm) up the side of the pan. (The water will help prevent the beets from drying out.) Cover and bake for 45 to 50 minutes, until the beets are fork-tender.

3. Meanwhile, roast the garlic. Remove the outer skin of the bulb and cut ¼ to ½ inch (5 mm to 1 cm) off the top of the cloves to expose the garlic. Place the garlic bulb cut side up on a small sheet of foil, drizzle with ½ teaspoon (2 mL) of the olive oil and let the oil seep into the garlic. Fold the foil over the garlic, sealing the package, and bake with the beets for 35 to 40 minutes, until the garlic is fork-tender.

4. Let the beets and garlic cool slightly. In a high-speed blender, combine the beets and garlic, remaining ¼ cup (60 mL) olive oil, tahini, rosemary and sea salt. Blend until smooth.

5. Scrape into a serving bowl. Just before serving, garnish with the sesame seeds and a drizzle of olive oil. Store leftovers in an airtight container in the fridge for up to 1 week.

Cauliflower Hummus
Dairy-free • Gluten-free • Grain-free • Kid-friendly • Vegan

Makes 2 cups (500 mL)

Every so often I need a break from traditional chickpea hummus because in our home, we eat a lot of this stuff. There are no chickpeas in this recipe, but it's just as fulfilling and creamy. Cauliflower is the main ingredient here, but if you suspect it won't be as tasty, think again! This low-carb, bean-free hummus is so delicious you may actually prefer it to the traditional kind.

If you have the time and want to take this recipe to a whole new level, I recommend roasting the garlic because it sweetens and mellows the taste (see page 77 for instructions on roasting garlic). And if you're strapped for time, instead of roasting the cauliflower, you could boil it for 5 to 7 minutes, until it's fork-tender. However, it will not be as flavourful. This dip is absolutely delicious with a platter of crunchy raw vegetables and my Rosemary Beet Chips (page 81).

1 medium head cauliflower, roughly chopped
1 tablespoon (15 mL) + ¼ cup (60 mL) extra-virgin olive oil, divided, more for serving
Pinch of sea salt
1 to 2 cloves garlic
¼ cup (60 mL) tahini
Juice of 1 lemon
1 to 2 tablespoons (15 to 30 mL) filtered water, for desired consistency
¼ cup (60 mL) pine nuts

1. Preheat the oven to 350°F (180°C). Line 2 baking sheets with parchment paper.

2. Spread the cauliflower on one of the prepared baking sheets. Drizzle with 1 tablespoon (15 mL) of the olive oil and sprinkle with the sea salt; toss to combine. Bake for 20 to 25 minutes, until golden and fork-tender. A little bit of browning is fine, but be careful not to burn the cauliflower. If it's burning, reduce the oven temperature and cook for a little longer.

3. Let the cauliflower cool slightly and then transfer to a food processor or blender. Add the garlic, tahini, lemon juice and the remaining ¼ cup (60 mL) olive oil. Blend until smooth. If you want a thinner consistency, add water 1 tablespoon (15 mL) at a time.

4. Meanwhile, increase the oven temperature to 375°F (190°C). Spread the pine nuts on the second prepared baking sheet. Bake for 5 to 10 minutes, until lightly toasted and golden brown.

5. Just before serving, scrape the hummus into a serving bowl, drizzle with olive oil and top with the toasted pine nuts. Store leftovers in an airtight container in the fridge for up to 1 week.

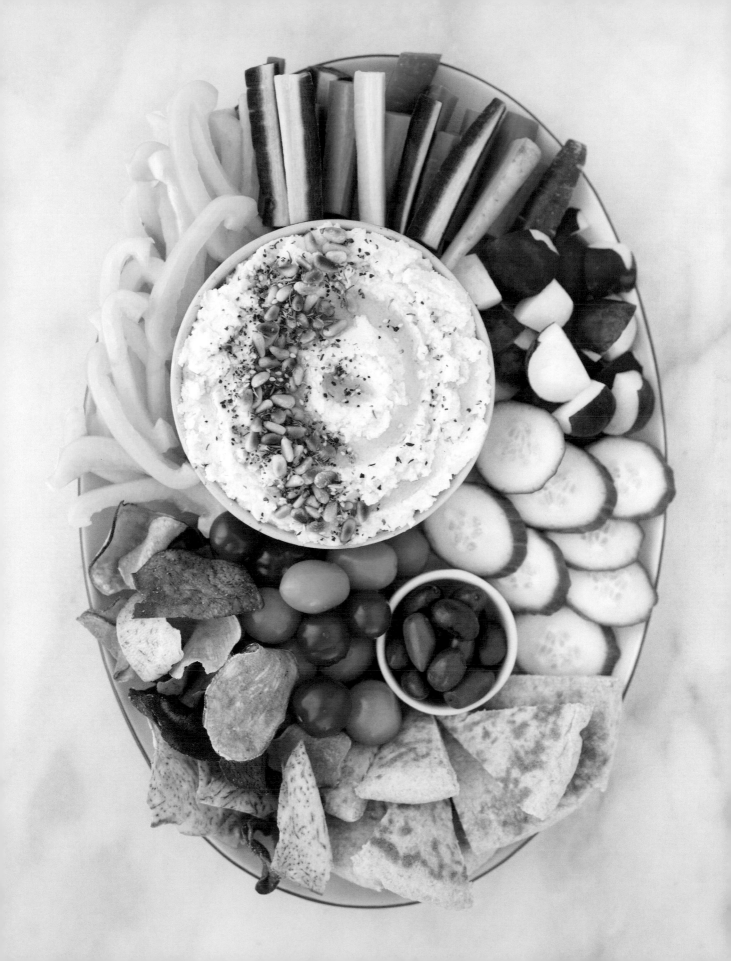

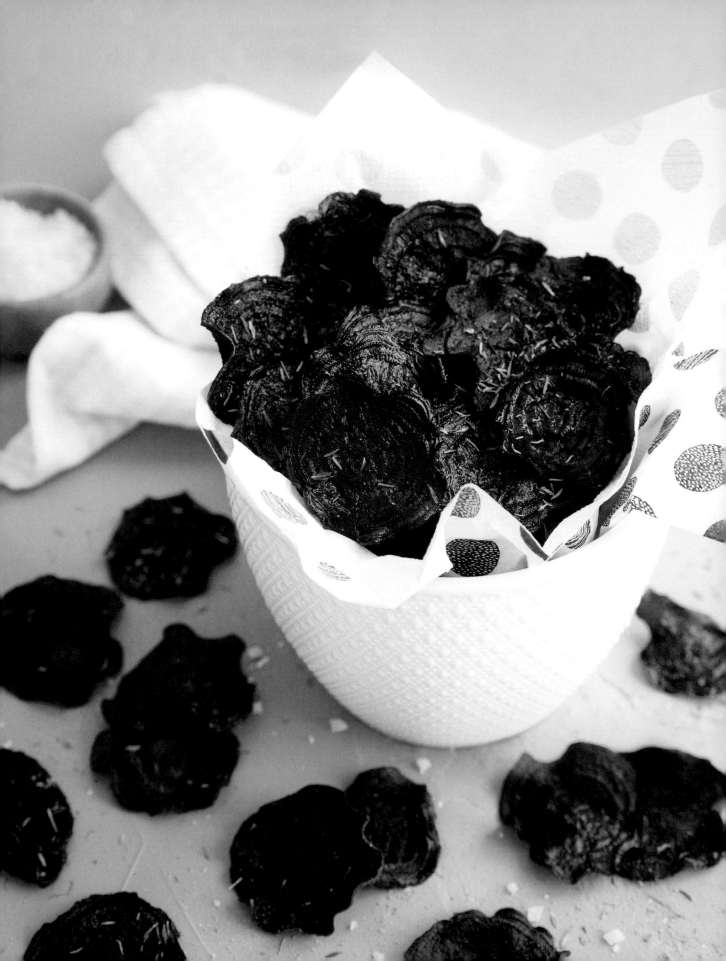

Rosemary Beet Chips

Dairy-free • Gluten-free • Grain-free • Kid-friendly • Nut-free • Vegan

Makes 3 cups (750 mL)

It's great that you can find root vegetable chips like beets and parsnips at most grocery stores, but the price prevents me from buying them regularly. Instead I make them at home. The homemade version tastes much better anyway!

I love a good salty snack, and when I need my fix, these beet chips are my go-to. They are a salty chip you can feel good about! The combination of rosemary, sea salt and beet is truly a match made in taste heaven. Be sure to store them only when they are completely cooled and crispy otherwise they will go soggy. Also, if you use too much olive oil they will stay too wet and then burn too fast. You'll need to watch the beet chips carefully to prevent burning. These go well with my Herby Tempeh Burgers (page 179).

3 medium red beets (unpeeled if organic),
   thinly sliced on a mandoline
1 teaspoon (5 mL) extra-virgin olive oil
1 teaspoon (5 mL) dried rosemary
¼ teaspoon (1 mL) sea salt

1. Preheat the oven to 400°F (200°C). Line a baking sheet with parchment paper.

2. Spread the beets evenly on the prepared baking sheet without overlapping. (You might need to bake them in two batches.) Drizzle lightly with olive oil and sprinkle with the rosemary and sea salt. Toss to coat and evenly spread on the baking sheet. Bake for 12 to 15 minutes, until the edges start to curl. Be careful because they can burn easily.

3. Cool completely on the baking sheet. Store in an airtight container at room temperature for up to 1 week.

Sun-Dried Tomato Olive Bread

Dairy-free • Kid-friendly • Vegetarian

Makes 1 loaf

Say goodbye to boring dinner rolls forever! This richly satisfying bread is perfect alongside my Creamy Kale and Apricot Salad with Roasted Chickpeas (page 107) or to smash an afternoon carb craving smothered with Original Ghee (page 43). The combination of sun-dried tomatoes and olives adds just the right amount of saltiness and heartiness, making this loaf one that I come back to again and again. In the middle of winter I absolutely love this loaf with a warm bowl of my Creamy Cremini Mushroom Soup (page 144).

½ cup (125 mL) pitted and chopped black olives

½ cup (125 mL) chopped sun-dried tomatoes in oil, drained

2 cups (500 mL) spelt flour

3 tablespoons (45 mL) nutritional yeast

1 tablespoon (15 mL) Italian seasoning

2 teaspoons (10 mL) baking powder

½ teaspoon (2 mL) baking soda

½ teaspoon (2 mL) sea salt

5 eggs

½ cup (125 mL) unsweetened almond milk

2 tablespoons + 1½ teaspoons (37 mL) olive oil

1. Preheat the oven to 350°F (180°C). Grease an 8½- × 4½-inch (1.5 L) loaf pan or line with parchment paper.

2. In a small bowl, mix together the olives and sun-dried tomatoes.

3. In a medium bowl, whisk together the spelt flour, nutritional yeast, Italian seasoning, baking powder, baking soda and sea salt.

4. In another medium bowl, whisk together the eggs, almond milk and olive oil. Add the wet mixture to the dry mixture and stir until combined. Fold in the olive mixture.

5. Scrape the batter into the prepared loaf pan and smooth the top. Bake for about 40 minutes, until a toothpick inserted in the centre of the loaf comes out clean.

6. Let cool in the pan for 10 minutes, then turn out onto a rack to cool for at least another 10 minutes before slicing. Store in an airtight container in the fridge for up to 1 week or slice, wrap individually and freeze in a resealable plastic freezer bag for up to 3 months.

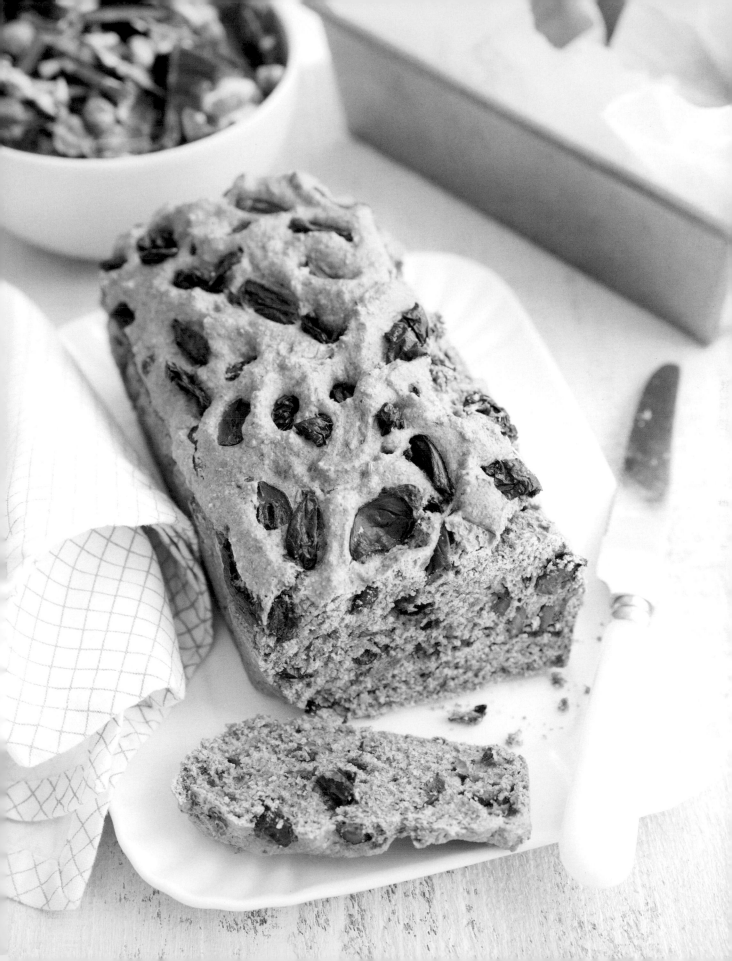

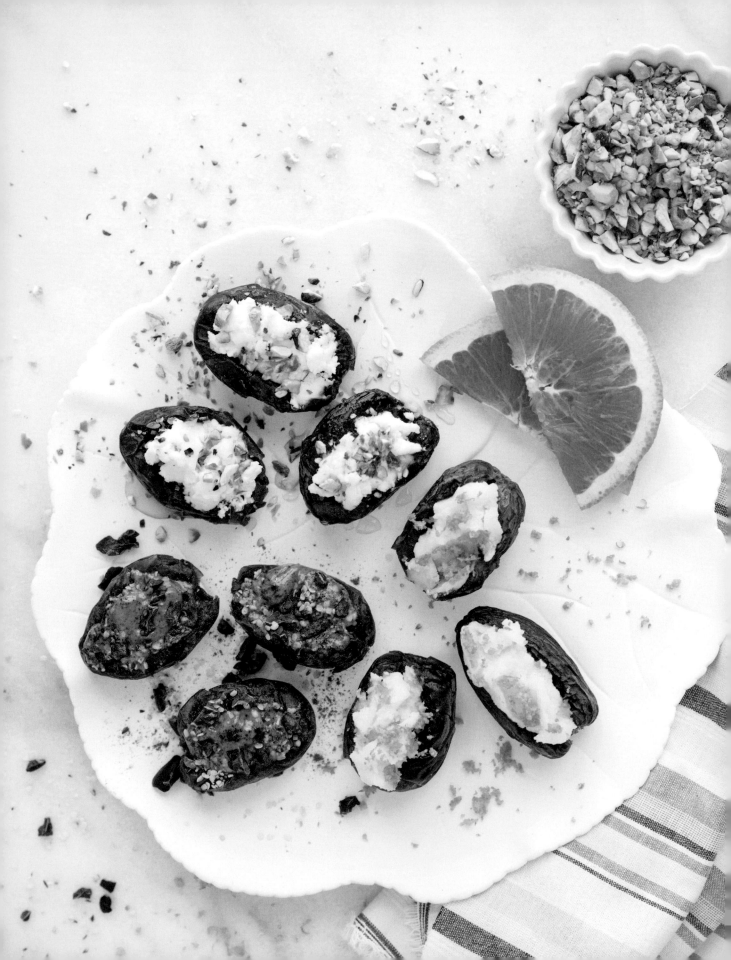

Stuffed Dates Three Ways

Each variation makes 6 dates

For the first twenty-five years of my life, the only dates I knew were puréed and added to date squares. Never in my wildest dreams would I ever have imagined I would be stuffing a date and eating it whole—that was such a foreign concept to me. However, times have changed!

These stuffed dates are a quick and naturally sweet snack that hits the spot when I've got a growl in my belly or a hankering for something sweet. I make them a variety of ways, but these three options are the most popular with my crowd. The Goat Cheese Pistachio Dates are the perfect appetizer to serve to guests, and the Almond Butter Chocolate Dates are a quick and easy dessert.

Coconut Orange Dates

Dairy-free • Gluten-free • Grain-free • Kid-friendly • Nut-free • Vegan

6 Medjool dates, pitted
1 tablespoon (15 mL) coconut butter
1 teaspoon (5 mL) freshly squeezed
   orange juice
1 teaspoon (5 mL) orange zest

1. In a small pot, gently warm the coconut butter over low heat. Stir in the orange juice.

2. Spoon the coconut butter mixture into the dates and top with orange zest. Enjoy immediately or refrigerate for 2 hours and enjoy them chilled. Store in an airtight container in the fridge for up to 5 days.

Almond Butter Chocolate Dates

Dairy-free • Gluten-free • Grain-free • Kid-friendly • Vegan

6 Medjool dates, pitted
1 tablespoon (15 mL) natural almond butter
1 teaspoon (5 mL) raw cacao nibs
1 teaspoon (5 mL) hemp seeds
½ teaspoon (2 mL) cinnamon

1. Spoon the almond butter into the dates.

2. Just before serving, top with raw cacao nibs, hemp seeds and a sprinkle of cinnamon. Store in an airtight container in the fridge for up to 5 days.

Goat Cheese Pistachio Dates

Gluten-free • Grain-free • Vegetarian

6 Medjool dates, pitted
1 tablespoon (15 mL) soft goat cheese
1 teaspoon (5 mL) finely chopped
   raw pistachios
Drizzle of pure liquid honey

1. Spoon the goat cheese into the dates.

2. Just before serving, top with pistachios and drizzle with honey. Store in an airtight container in the fridge for up to 5 days.

Oat, Spice and Everything Nice Balls

Dairy-free • Kid-friendly • Vegan

Makes 30 balls

Everyone loves these balls! The flavour combination of cinnamon, cardamom and nutmeg is really memorable. As well, those spices are super rich in antioxidants. These balls are more dense than your typical raw cookie ball because of the oats. Oats are rich in fibre, both soluble and insoluble, which is why they keep you nice and full as a power snack. They are also rich in resistant starch, which feeds the friendly bacteria that live in your digestive tract.

Enjoy a ball or two with my Green Mojito Smoothie (page 55) or for dessert after the Sweet Potato, Kale and Brown Rice Salad (page 108) for a delicious plant-based meal.

1 cup (250 mL) raw cashews
½ cup (125 mL) oat flakes or quick-cooking rolled oats
½ cup (125 mL) unsweetened shredded coconut
½ cup (125 mL) natural almond butter
12 Medjool dates, pitted
2 teaspoons (10 mL) cinnamon
½ teaspoon (2 mL) ground cardamom
½ teaspoon (2 mL) ground nutmeg
1 tablespoon (15 mL) filtered water, for desired consistency

1. Place all the ingredients, except the water, in a food processor. Process for 45 to 60 seconds, until the mixture is crumbly. If the mixture is too dry, add water as needed.

2. Using your hands, roll the mixture into 1- inch (2.5 cm) balls. Store in an airtight container in the fridge for up to 2 weeks or in the freezer for up 3 months.

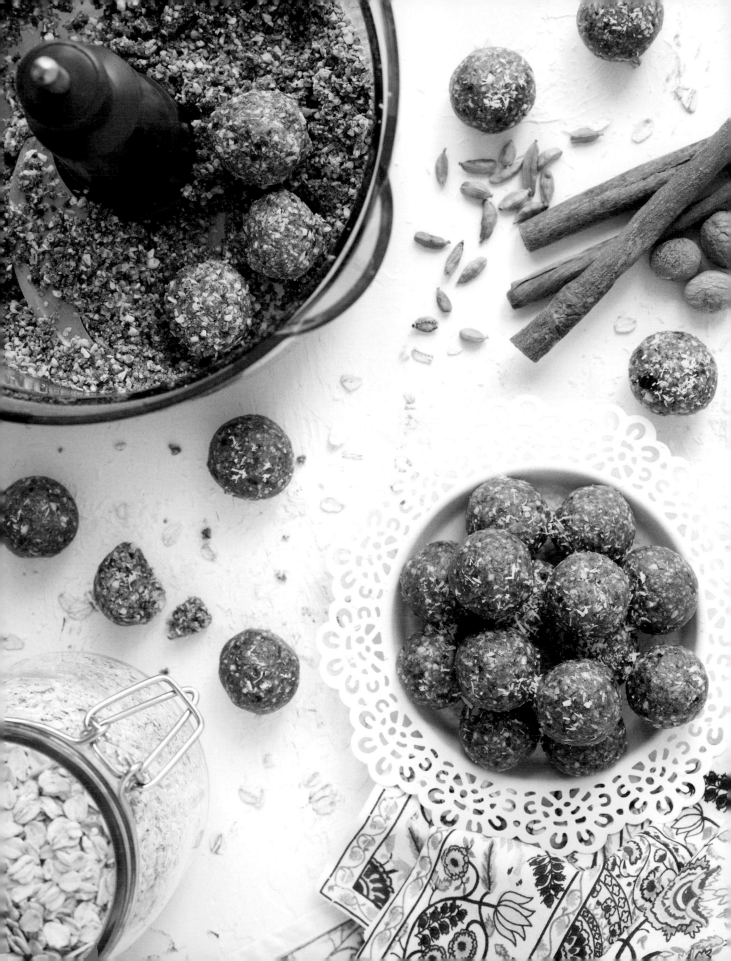

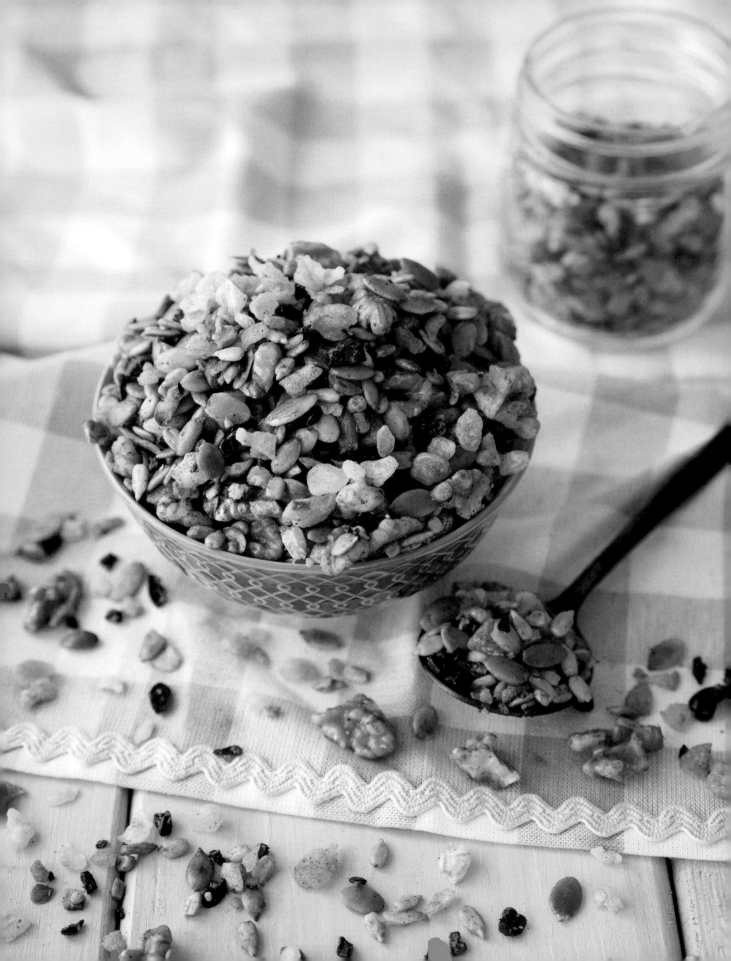

Picnic Trail Mix

Dairy-free • Gluten-free • Grain-free • Kid-friendly • Vegan

Makes 2½ cups (625 mL)

Trail mix is something I always keep stocked in our home. Whenever I have the midday munchies, a handful of this mix saves me from eating the whole batch of Rosemary Beet Chips (page 81) or all the Dark Chocolate Superfood Bars (page 224)! Whether you're picnicking or not, trail mix is an energizing snack. It has plenty of plant-based protein and good fats to keep your blood sugar balanced and your belly satisfied for hours. This trail mix satisfies both sweet and salty cravings.

The hero of this recipe is definitely the crystallized ginger, which you'll find at bulk food stores. If you don't have walnuts, pumpkin seeds or sunflower seeds on hand, any other nut or seed will do.

1 tablespoon (15 mL) coconut oil
½ teaspoon (2 mL) cinnamon
¼ teaspoon (1 mL) ground nutmeg
Pinch of sea salt
1 cup (250 mL) whole raw walnuts
½ cup (125 mL) raw pumpkin seeds
½ cup (125 mL) raw sunflower seeds
¼ cup (60 mL) raw cacao nibs
¼ cup (60 mL) chopped crystalized ginger

1. In a small pot, melt the coconut oil over low heat. Add the cinnamon, nutmeg and sea salt and stir. Remove from the heat.

2. In a large bowl, combine the walnuts, pumpkin seeds, sunflower seeds, cacao nibs and ginger. Pour the coconut oil mixture over the nut and seed mixture and stir to evenly coat. Store in an airtight container, preferably a mason jar, for up to 4 weeks.

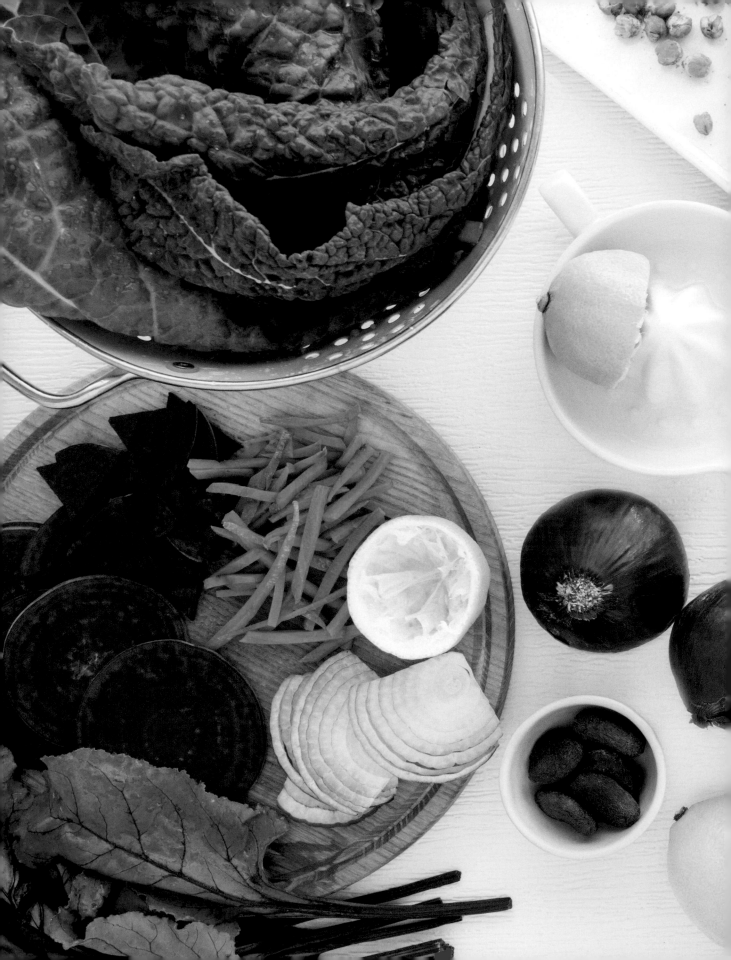

Salads and Sides

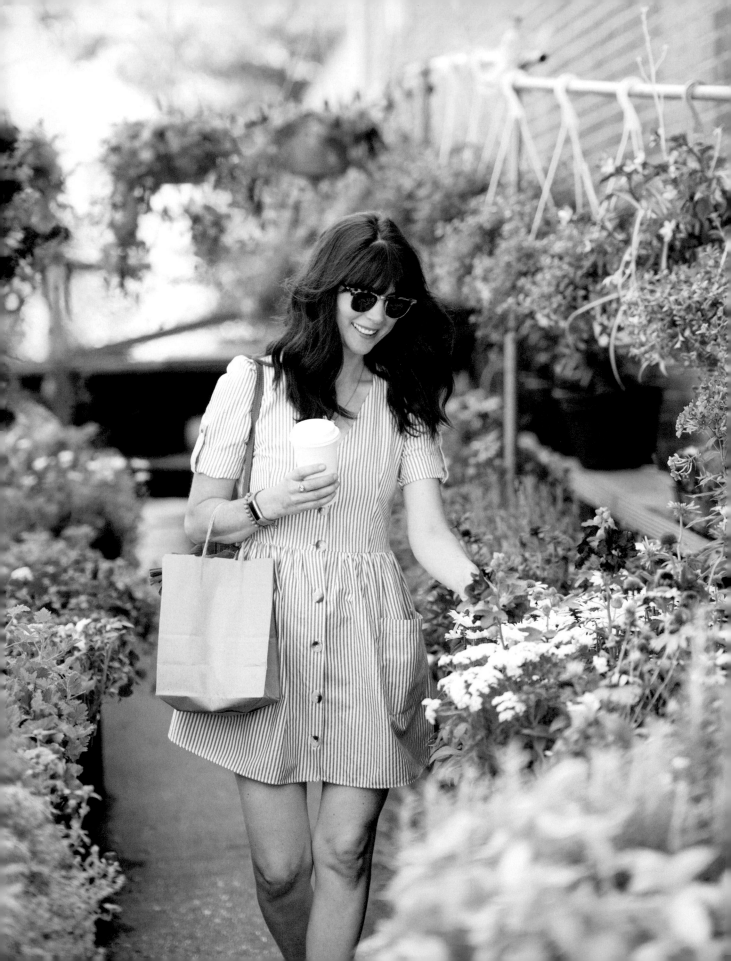

SALADS AND SIDES

I eat a lot of salads and sides. In fact, I've been known to eat a whole meal of just sides. I mean, how could you resist a plate of my Crunchy Beet and Carrot Quinoa Salad (page 103) alongside my Broccoli and Cranberry Salad with Creamy Dill Dressing (page 104)? Given the right ingredients, sides absolutely satisfy me both emotionally and physically. Throughout the year I eat salads, but the ingredients change depending on the season and availability. In the summer and into early fall I prefer more raw salads, such as my Shredded Brussels Sprouts Bean Salad with Honey ACV Dressing (page 100). In the winter, I prefer more comforting salads with roasted vegetables, like my Sweet Potato, Kale and Brown Rice Salad (page 108). I could eat salad 365 days a year because I love the way my body feels when I eat lots of plant-based foods.

The key to a satisfying salad is an epic dressing that you'll want to drizzle on everything. A salad dressing should not be boring! Some salads and sides can be meals on their own if you use hearty ingredients with a balance of satiating good fat and protein. Or they can complement another dish, like a soup. My Za'atar Socca (page 130) goes amazingly well with the Creamy Cremini Mushroom Soup (page 144) for a fulfilling and flavourful lunch or dinner. One thing's for sure, every salad or side in this chapter is keeping you on or getting you onto the path to your most joyous health ever.

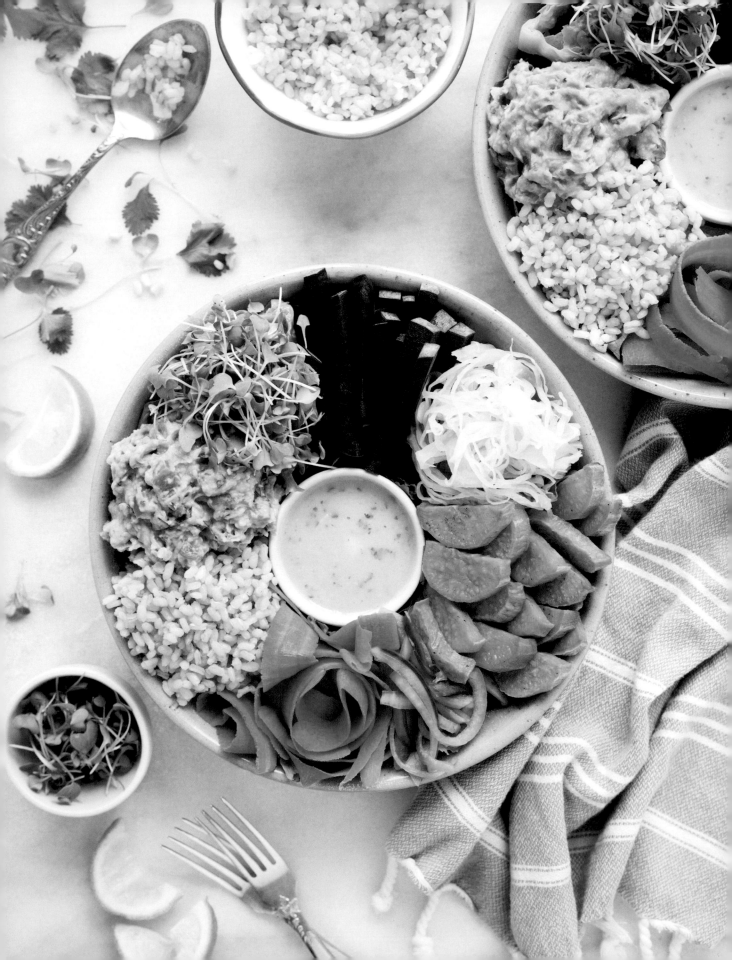

Hungry Gal Buddha Bowl

Dairy-free • Gluten-free • Nut-free • Vegan

Serves 2

This is the salad bowl that Instagram dreams are made of! It's super filling because of all that fibre and healthy fat and it's amazing for gut health as well thanks to the sauerkraut, pickled onions and broccoli sprouts. However, don't let the photo intimidate you. If you have an extra ten minutes to beautify it, then by all means go for it. If not, just toss everything together like I usually do. It's just as delicious all mixed together.

Normally I keep my salad dressings simple, using either tahini and lemon juice or olive oil and apple cider vinegar. But sometimes I feel like having something a little more creamy that still has a nice bright flavour. This Avocado Lime Dressing is so versatile, you'll be making it for all your salads whenever you have perfectly ripe avocados. Whenever I'm baking sweet potatoes for dinner, I toss in a few extras, just so I have leftovers for dishes like this.

Avocado Lime Dressing

½ large ripe avocado, pitted, peeled and roughly chopped
½ cup (125 mL) loosely packed fresh cilantro or basil leaves
Juice of 2 limes
1 or 2 cloves garlic
¼ cup (60 mL) extra-virgin olive oil
3 tablespoons (45 mL) filtered water

Buddha Bowl

1 cup (250 mL) Ginger Sesame Guacamole (page 73)
1 large red beet (unpeeled if organic), cut into matchsticks
2 carrots, grated or peeled into ribbons
6 tablespoons (90 mL) sauerkraut
¼ cup (60 mL) Quick Pickled Onions (page 133)
1 sweet potato, baked, sliced into rounds or cut into cubes
6 tablespoons (90 mL) broccoli sprouts
1 cup (250 mL) cooked brown rice
4 cups (1 L) chopped romaine lettuce or kale

1. **Make the Avocado Lime Dressing** Place the avocado, cilantro, lime juice, garlic, olive oil and water in a food processor or high-speed blender. Blend until smooth. Store in an airtight container in the fridge for up to 3 days.

2. **Assemble the Buddha Bowls** Divide the ingredients evenly between 2 bowls, assembling in segments or just tossing all the ingredients together. Drizzle the dressing over the salad. Enjoy immediately.

Summer Salad with Halloumi

Gluten-free • Grain-free • Nut-free • Vegetarian

Serves 4

I discovered halloumi cheese at a Middle Eastern restaurant. I later found it at my local grocery store. Now I buy it every week throughout the summer from my local farmers' market, just so I can make this salad. I absolutely love halloumi. It's one of my favourite salty foods.

   Most halloumi cheese is made from sheeps' or goat milk and some is made from cow's milk. It's salty and absolutely delicious when you warm it up in a frying pan. If you can't find halloumi, you can use feta or a firm goat cheese instead. You can likely find all the salad ingredients local and organic—the best of both worlds! This salad goes great with the summery fresh taste of my Chilled Zucchini Avocado Basil Soup (page 139).

Summer Salad

5 cups (1.25 L) tightly packed fresh arugula

2 cups (500 mL) fresh strawberries, chopped

3 carrots, very thinly sliced into ribbons

½ small red onion, finely chopped

½ English cucumber, cut in half lengthwise and sliced in half-moons

6 radishes, thinly sliced

9 ounces (250 g) halloumi cheese, cut into 8 slices (¼ inch/5 mm thick)

Dijon Maple Dressing

½ cup (125 mL) extra-virgin olive oil

2 tablespoons (30 mL) Dijon mustard

2 tablespoons (30 mL) real maple syrup

1 clove garlic, minced

2 tablespoons (30 mL) filtered water

1. **Make the Summer Salad** In a large salad bowl, toss together the arugula, strawberries, carrots, red onion, cucumber and radishes.

2. **Make the Dijon Maple Dressing** In a small bowl, whisk together the olive oil, mustard, maple syrup, garlic and water until emulsified.

3. Heat a frying pan over medium heat. Fry the halloumi slices until golden brown on the bottom, about 5 minutes. Flip and continue cooking until golden brown, 2 to 3 minutes.

4. To serve, drizzle the dressing over the salad and top with the halloumi. Enjoy immediately.

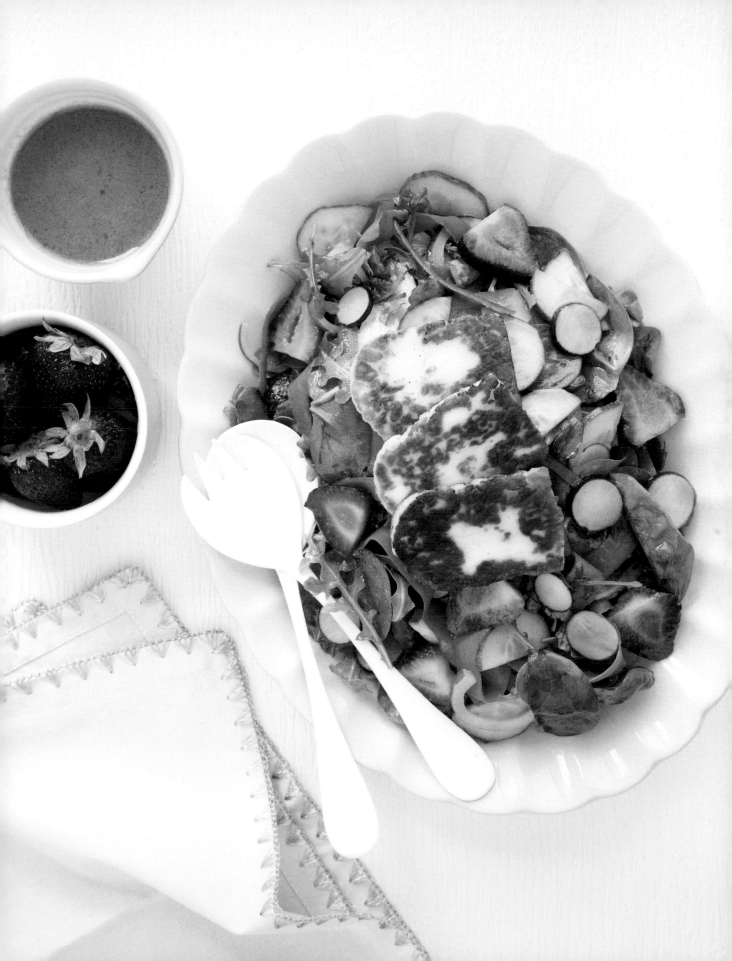

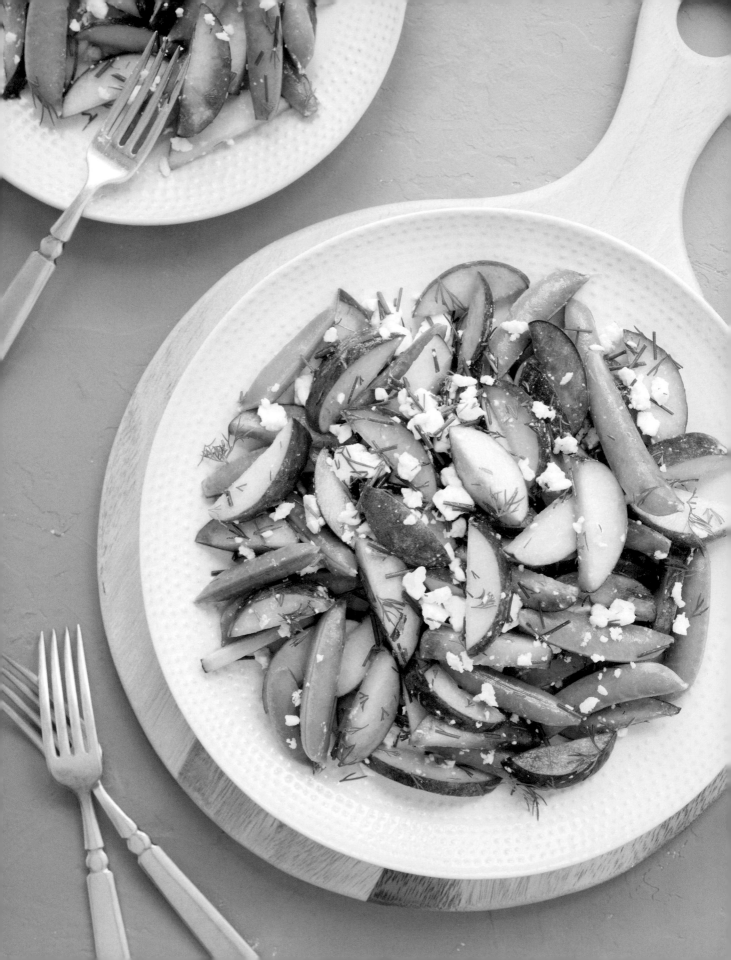

Peach and Snap Pea Salad

Gluten-free • Grain-free • Kid-friendly • Nut-free • Vegetarian

Serves 4

Every summer I eat my weight in peaches! I just can't help it, they are the perfect fruit—juicy, sweet and incredibly versatile because they work in both sweet and savoury dishes. When they are in season, we pick up at least two baskets on our weekly farmers' market visits. On the way back home we each end up eating two peaches.

   I used to think of peaches only in sweet dishes until an amazing lunch I had at a hotel in Lake Louise, Alberta. They used local peaches and combined them with feta and snap peas. This inspired me to create this wonderful peach salad with local herbs. It is fragrant and flavourful!

6 ripe firm peaches, pitted and chopped into bite-size chunks
1 cup (250 mL) sugar snap peas
2 tablespoons (30 mL) chopped fresh chives
2 tablespoons (30 mL) chopped fresh dill
Juice of ½ lemon
1 tablespoon (15 mL) extra-virgin olive oil
½ cup (125 mL) crumbled sheep's milk feta cheese

1. In a large salad bowl, combine the peaches, snap peas, chives and dill.

2. Drizzle with the lemon juice and olive oil, then toss. Top with the feta and enjoy immediately.

Shredded Brussels Sprouts Bean Salad with Honey ACV Dressing

Dairy-free • Gluten-free • Grain-free • Nut-free • Vegetarian

Serves 6

Whenever I'm travelling, I still eat healthy, but if I'm cooking in a kitchen with the bare essentials (a bar fridge and a tiny counter), I make sure the meals I create are simple. I always visit the local health food store and pick up packages of shredded Brussels sprouts and grated carrots, which makes the prep work faster and easier. Then I chop the remaining ingredients. If you want to save some money and you've got a little more time on your hands, then doing the prep of the veggies is well worth the effort. To speed up the process, run the Brussels sprouts, carrots and apple through a food processor fitted with the shredding disc or "S" blade, it works with both.

The dressing is fresh and bright, and the crunchiness of this salad will keep you coming back for more. I love eating this salad for lunch, as it makes a whole meal and it's super satisfying.

Shredded Brussels Sprouts Bean Salad

5 cups (1.25 L) shredded Brussels sprouts
2 cups (500 mL) grated carrots
2 cups (500 mL) grated apple
½ cup (125 mL) dried cranberries
3 shallots (or 1 small red onion),
  finely chopped
1 can (15 ounces/425 g) navy beans,
  drained and rinsed
Sprinkle of sea salt
3 tablespoons (45 mL) chopped fresh
  mint, for garnish

Honey ACV Dressing

⅔ cup (150 mL) extra-virgin olive oil
½ cup (125 mL) raw apple cider vinegar
2 tablespoons (30 mL) pure liquid honey
1 clove garlic, minced

1. Make the Shredded Brussels Sprouts Bean Salad In a large bowl, combine the Brussels sprouts, carrots, apple, cranberries, shallots and navy beans. Toss well. Store in an airtight container in the fridge for up to 3 days.

2. Make the Honey ACV Dressing In a small bowl, whisk together the olive oil, apple cider vinegar, honey and garlic until emulsified.

3. Pour the dressing over the salad and toss. Sprinkle the sea salt on top. Garnish with the mint and serve.

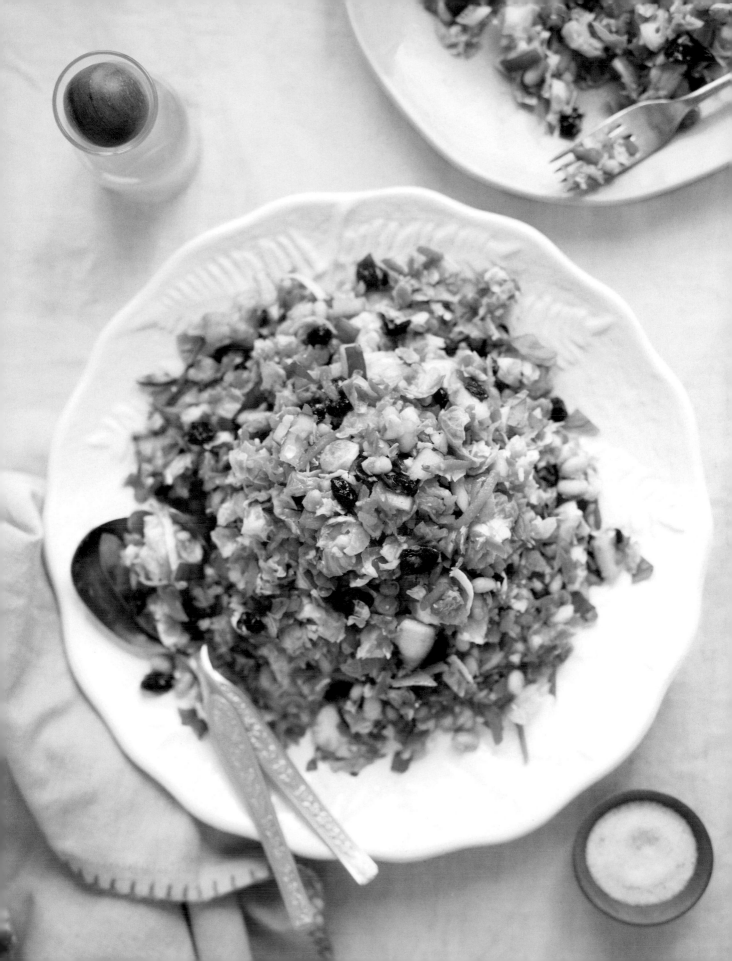

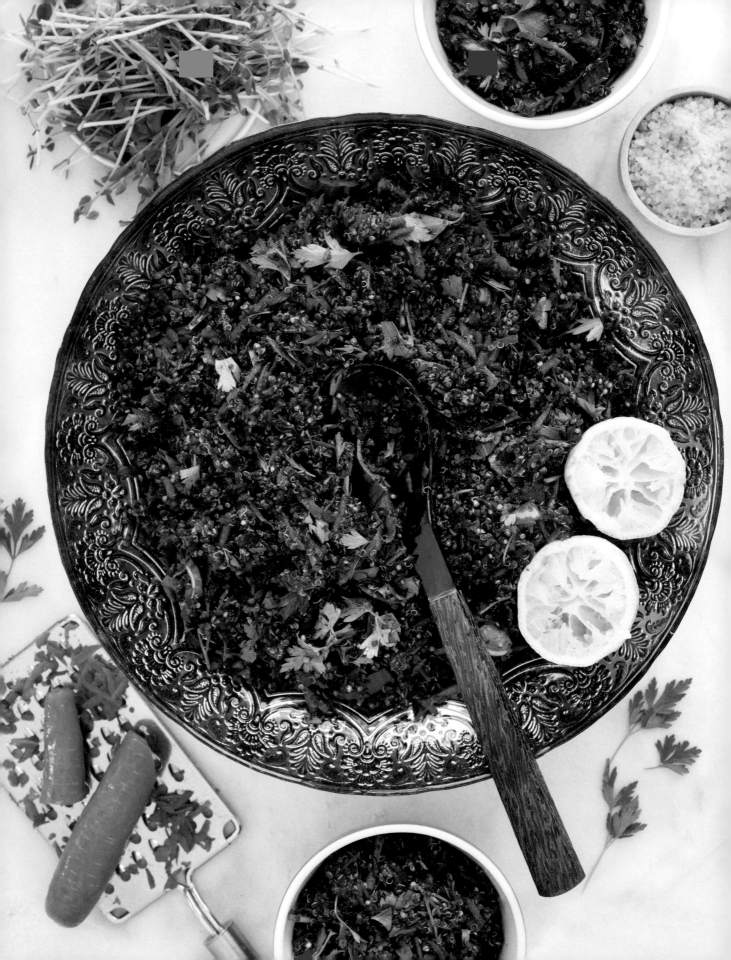

Crunchy Beet and Carrot Quinoa Salad

Dairy-free • Gluten-free • Kid-friendly • Nut-free • Vegan

Serves 4

I love a good crunch when I'm eating a meal. It makes me feel like I'm eating something with substance and it's more satisfying. Eating this salad also reminds me to be mindful when eating, because you can't eat it quickly: you've really gotta chew! As a nutritionist, I'm always harping on the fact that it is important to eat slowly and chew our food thoroughly for better digestion. As soon as my daughter had more teeth, she got into this salad too. It shocked Walker and me that a toddler would enjoy this salad, but we didn't question it. We just smiled!

We love this salad alongside Herby Tempeh Burgers (page 179) or the Super-Quick Tortilla Pizzas (page 175).

Crunchy Beet and Carrot Quinoa Salad

1 cup (250 mL) white quinoa
2 cups (500 mL) water
2 cups (500 mL) grated carrots
2 cups (500 mL) finely chopped
 or grated beets
½ medium red onion, finely chopped
1 cup (250 mL) loosely packed chopped
 fresh curly or flat-leaf parsley
Pea sprouts, for garnish

Lemon Olive Oil Dressing

Juice of 2 lemons
⅓ cup (75 mL) extra-virgin olive oil
Sea salt

1. **Make the Crunchy Beet and Carrot Quinoa Salad** Combine the quinoa and water in a small saucepan and bring to a boil. Reduce the heat and simmer, with the lid slightly ajar, for 15 minutes, or until fluffy. Remove from the heat and cool completely.

2. Meanwhile, in a large salad bowl, combine the carrots, beets, red onion and parsley. Stir in the cooked quinoa.

3. **Make the Lemon Olive Oil Dressing** In a small bowl, whisk together the lemon juice, olive oil and sea salt to taste until emulsified.

4. Pour the dressing over the salad, top with pea sprouts and serve immediately. Alternatively, you can store the salad (with the dressing) in the fridge until ready to serve, then top with pea sprouts.

Broccoli and Cranberry Salad with Creamy Dill Dressing

Gluten-free • Grain-free • Kid-friendly • Vegetarian

Serves 4

I make this salad for family gatherings because kids and grown-ups alike always love the mixture of ingredients. Parents are happy because their kids are eating broccoli, and kids are happy because it tastes yummy! It's a total crowd-pleaser.

You can easily make this dairy-free by using coconut yogurt or cashew yogurt. Just make sure it's unsweetened. I really love the sour taste of plain sheep's milk yogurt, and nowadays it's pretty easy to find at most health food stores and in the natural foods section of big grocery stores. I like to serve this with my Rustic Mediterranean Summer Galette (page 199). And for dessert, the Almond Butter Rice Crispy Squares (page 220) are perfect.

Broccoli and Cranberry Salad

6 cups (1.5 L) broccoli florets
½ medium red onion, thinly sliced
½ cup (125 mL) roughly chopped
    raw cashews or almonds
½ cup (125 mL) dried cranberries

Creamy Dill Dressing

1 cup (250 mL) unsweetened plain full-fat
    sheep's yogurt or coconut yogurt
¼ cup (60 mL) lemon juice
2 tablespoons (30 mL) chopped fresh dill
1 teaspoon (5 mL) garlic powder
1 teaspoon (5 mL) apple cider vinegar
    or white wine vinegar
½ teaspoon (2 mL) sea salt

1. **Prepare the broccoli** Bring a large pot of water to a boil. Add the broccoli and cook for 2 to 3 minutes, until crisp-tender and bright green. Drain the broccoli and rinse in cold water. Place in a large bowl and chill in the fridge while you make the dressing.

2. **Meanwhile, make the Creamy Dill Dressing** In a small bowl, whisk together the yogurt, lemon juice, dill, garlic powder, apple cider vinegar and sea salt.

3. **Assemble the Broccoli and Cranberry Salad** To the broccoli, add the red onion, cashews and cranberries. Pour the dressing over the salad and toss. Refrigerate until ready to serve. This salad is best served the day it is made or it gets soggy.

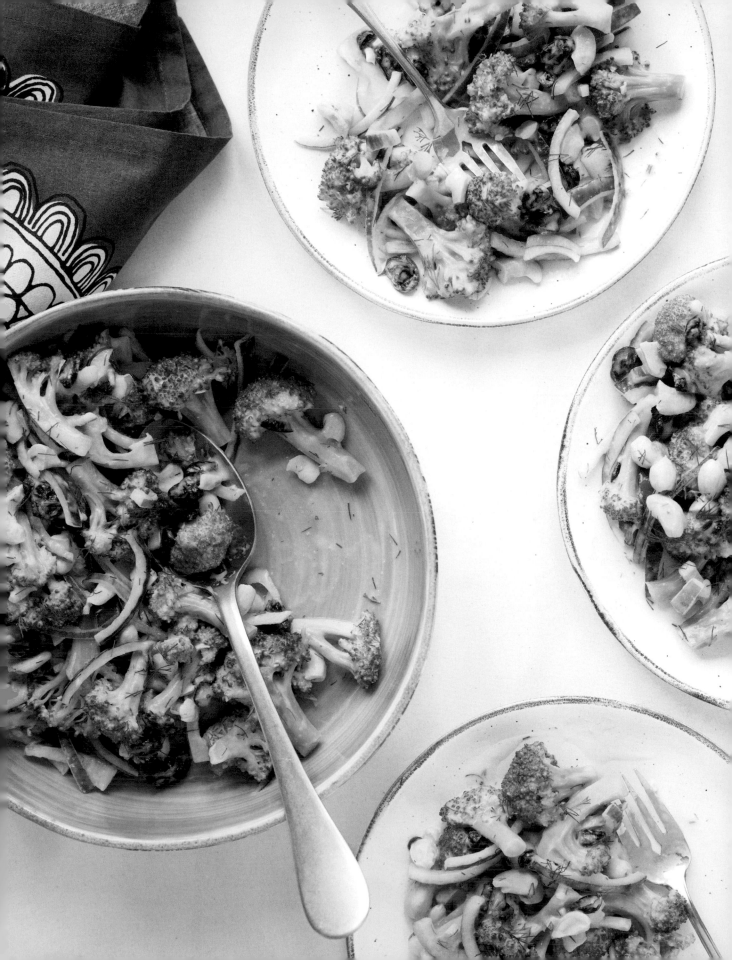

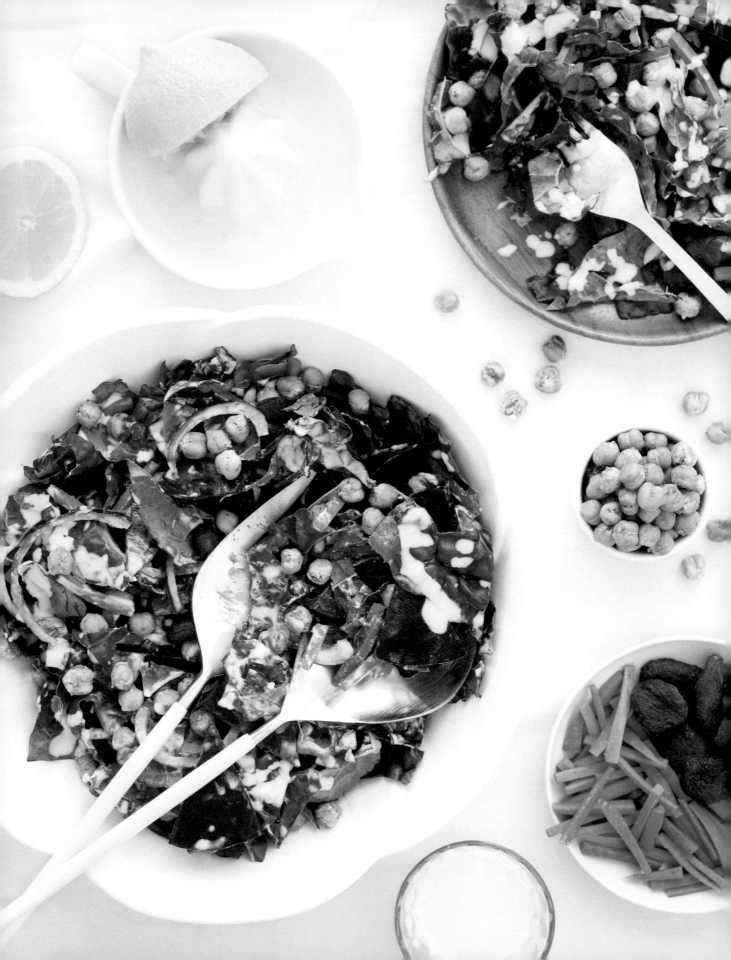

Creamy Kale and Apricot Salad with Roasted Chickpeas

Dairy-free • Gluten-free • Grain-free • Kid-friendly • Nut-free • Vegan

Serves 4

This is a beloved recipe from my *Joyous Health* blog that I have made more times than I can count. The combination of creaminess from the dressing and the crunchy raw salad and chickpeas is pure pleasure! Roasted chickpeas are a favourite with my family because they are crunchy, salty and packed with plant-based protein and fibre. This is a meat-free meal that is just as satisfying as eating a piece of grilled chicken or fish.

If there are only small bunches of kale at the grocery store or farmers' market, then use two for this recipe. For a generous serving of salad, I measure how much kale I need based on two large handfuls of chopped kale per person. To slice the beets nice and thin, use a mandoline if you have one. Make sure the dried apricots you're using are brown, as this means they are free of preservatives like sulphites. If your crowd is hungry, this salad goes nicely with my Zucchini Fritters (page 126).

Roasted Chickpeas

1 can (15 ounces/425 g) chickpeas, drained and rinsed
½ teaspoon (2 mL) garlic powder
½ teaspoon (2 mL) sweet paprika
½ teaspoon (2 mL) Italian seasoning

Kale Salad

1 to 2 bunches lacinato kale, centre stems removed, roughly chopped
2 medium red beets (unpeeled if organic), thinly sliced
1 cup (250 mL) carrot matchsticks or grated carrot
½ cup (125 mL) chopped dried unsulphured apricots
1 small red onion, finely chopped

Creamy Tahini Dressing

3 heaping tablespoons (54 mL) tahini
2 tablespoons (30 mL) extra-virgin olive oil
Juice of 1 lemon
1 to 2 cloves garlic, finely minced
Pinch of sea salt
Filtered water, just enough for desired consistency

1. **Make the Roasted Chickpeas** Preheat the oven to 350°F (180°C). Line a baking sheet with parchment paper.

2. Spread the chickpeas on a kitchen towel. Top with another kitchen towel and pat dry. This will help the spices stick to the chickpeas. Place the chickpeas in a medium bowl, sprinkle with the garlic powder, paprika and Italian seasoning, and toss to coat.

3. Evenly spread the chickpeas on the prepared baking sheet and bake for 35 to 40 minutes, until crispy and golden brown. If they are not crispy after 30 minutes, increase the heat to 375°F (190°C) and cook for 5 to 10 minutes longer—just be careful they don't burn. Set aside until you're ready to add them to the salad.

4. **Meanwhile, make the Kale Salad** In a large salad bowl, combine the kale, beets, carrots, apricots and red onion.

5. **Make the Creamy Tahini Dressing** In a small bowl, whisk together the tahini, olive oil, lemon juice, garlic and sea salt. Add water to thin the dressing, as needed. (I find a couple of tablespoons works nicely.)

6. Sprinkle the Roasted Chickpeas on top of the Kale Salad and drizzle with the Creamy Tahini Dressing. Store any leftover chickpeas in an airtight container at room temperature for up to 5 days.

Sweet Potato, Kale and Brown Rice Salad

Gluten-free • Kid-friendly • Nut-free • Vegetarian

Serves 4 to 6

I've been making a variation of this amazing salad for many years. No matter who I make it for, whether they are health nuts or not, everyone loves it. Nothing makes me happier than feeding my family and friends something they enjoy and seeing them go for seconds. The combination of brown rice, navy beans and greens makes this a real "stick to your ribs" dish but won't leave you feeling stuffed. The simple dressing has just the right amount of flavour to let the salad ingredients really shine.

This is a wonderful side dish to my Rosemary and Thyme Roasted Chicken with Baby Potatoes (page 165), or serve it on its own as a vegetarian main with Roasted Pear and Parsnip Soup with Kale Chips (page 147).

3 cups (750 mL) diced sweet potato

1 tablespoon (15 mL) + ⅓ cup (75 mL) extra-virgin olive oil, divided

Sea salt

1 cup (250 mL) brown rice

2 cups (500 mL) water

1 bunch curly kale, centre stems removed, chopped into bite-size pieces

1 small red onion, finely chopped

1 can (15 ounces /425 g) navy beans, drained and rinsed

½ cup (125 mL) dried cranberries

¼ cup (60 mL) loosely packed chopped fresh curly or flat-leaf parsley

Juice of 2 lemons

½ cup (125 mL) crumbled feta cheese

Pepper

1. Preheat the oven to 375°F (190°C). Line a baking sheet with parchment paper.

2. Evenly spread the sweet potatoes on the prepared baking sheet. Drizzle with 1 tablespoon (15 mL) of the olive oil and sprinkle with a pinch of sea salt. Bake for 25 to 30 minutes, until fork-tender.

3. In a medium pot, combine the brown rice and water. Bring to a boil over medium-high heat. Reduce the heat to a low simmer, cover and cook until the rice is tender and fluffs with a fork, 25 to 30 minutes.

4. In a large salad bowl, combine the kale, red onion, navy beans, cranberries and parsley. Add the cooked rice while still warm and mix together. If you are not serving the salad right away, store it in the fridge.

5. To make the dressing, whisk together the lemon juice and the remaining ⅓ cup (75 mL) olive oil until emulsified. Pour the dressing over the salad and toss. Top with the feta. Sprinkle with sea salt and pepper to taste.

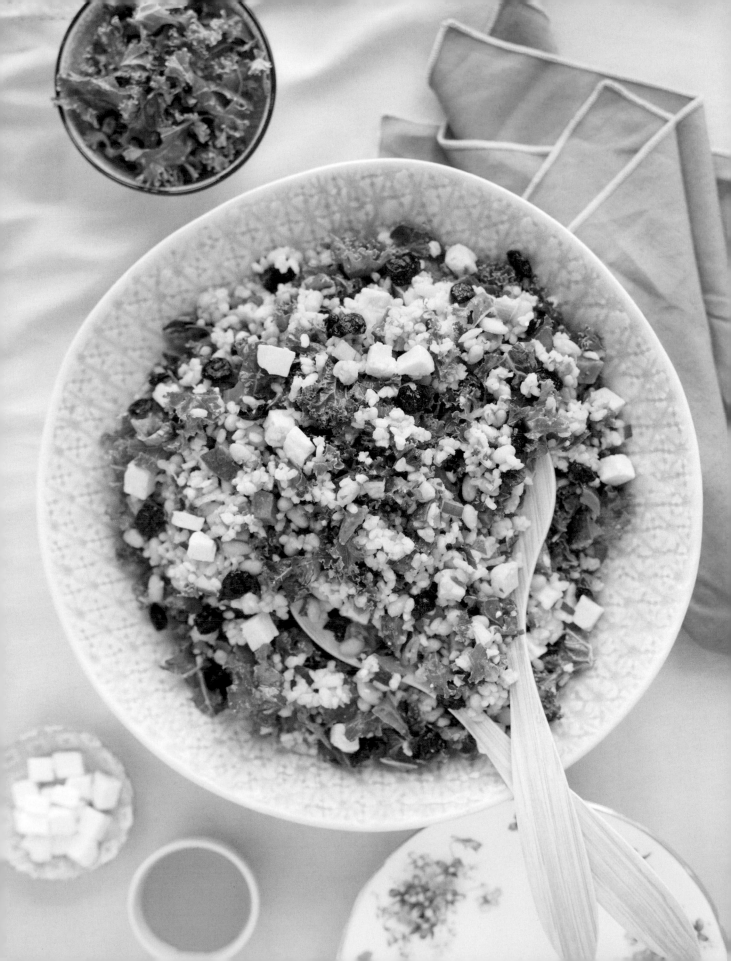

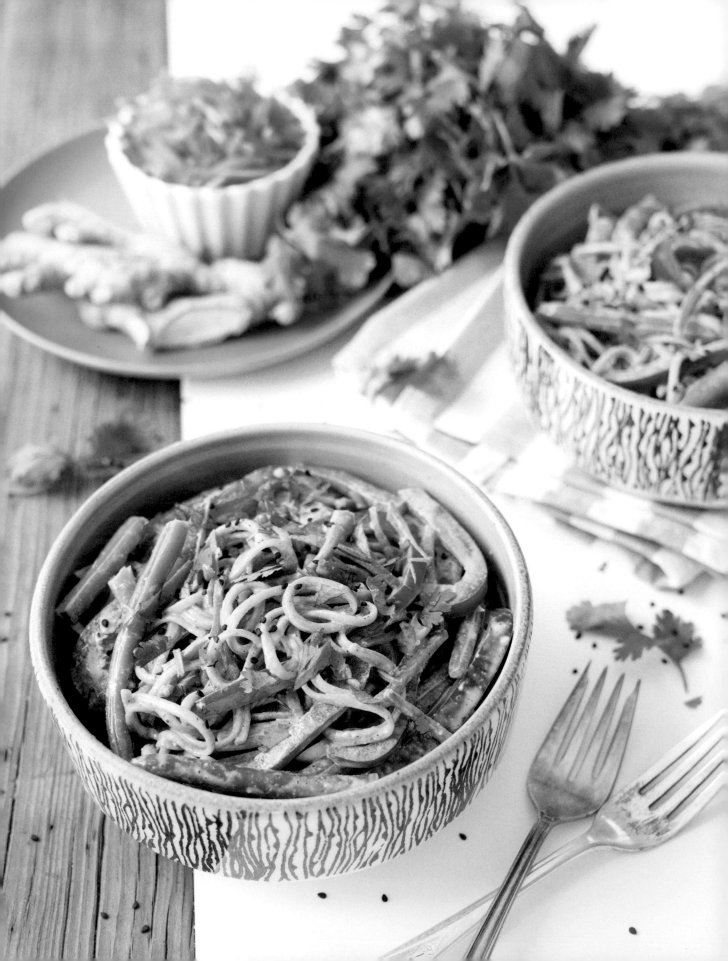

Crunchy and Creamy Soba Noodle Salad with Almond Dressing

Dairy-free • Gluten-free • Vegetarian

Serves 4 as a side, 2 as a main

Soba noodles are a favourite of mine because they cook so quickly and are a good source of protein, fibre and minerals. I use King Soba 100 percent organic buckwheat noodles in this recipe.

Crunchy and creamy, this soba noodle salad is satisfying to all the senses. The dressing is rich with good fat, making the salad a meal all on its own, or it goes well with some added protein, like my Lemon Pepper Baked Trout (page 203). You can leave out the chili flakes if you're making it for little ones, as I often do. If not, I highly recommend some heat. The chili flakes match so well with the richness of the dressing. You can skip blanching the green beans if you like: it's not necessary, and I like them crunchy. It's up to you!

Almond Dressing

¼ cup (60 mL) tahini
2 tablespoons (30 mL) natural almond butter
2 tablespoons (30 mL) gluten-free tamari
1 tablespoon (15 mL) toasted sesame oil
2 teaspoons (10 mL) grated fresh ginger
1 teaspoon (5 mL) pure liquid honey
1 teaspoon (5 mL) red chili flakes (optional)
1 clove garlic, minced
¼ cup (60 mL) filtered water

Crunchy and Creamy Soba Noodle Salad

2 cups (500 mL) green beans, trimmed
9 ounces (250 g) buckwheat soba noodles
1 sweet red pepper, cut into matchsticks
½ cup (125 mL) shredded carrot
¼ cup (60 mL) chopped green onions (white and light green parts only)

Garnish

¼ cup (60 mL) tightly packed chopped fresh cilantro
1 teaspoon (5 mL) red chili flakes (optional)
½ teaspoon (2 mL) black or white sesame seeds

1. **Make the Almond Dressing** In a small bowl, whisk together the tahini, almond butter, tamari, sesame oil, ginger, honey, chili flakes (if using), garlic and water.

2. **Make the Crunchy and Creamy Soba Noodle Salad** Bring a large pot of water to a boil. Prepare a medium bowl of ice water. Add the green beans to the boiling water and cook for 2 to 3 minutes, until crisp-tender. Using a slotted spoon, immediately transfer the green beans to the bowl of ice water to chill.

3. Return the water to a boil. Add the soba noodles and cook until just tender, 5 to 6 minutes or according to package directions. Drain the noodles and rinse under cold water. Drain well.

4. Drain the green beans and pat dry. Place the noodles in a large salad bowl and add the green beans, red pepper, carrots and green onions. Toss to combine. Pour the Almond Dressing over the salad and toss. Garnish with the cilantro, chili flakes (if using) and sesame seeds.

Baked Cauliflower and Broccoli with Tahini Lemon Sauce

Dairy-free • Gluten-free • Grain-free • Kid-friendly • Nut-free • Vegan

Serves 4

This dish is on repeat in our home because we have a veggie-loving daughter, and two of her favourites are cauliflower and broccoli. If you're trying to get someone—child or adult—to eat more veggies, this dish is a good place to start. The salty olive oil drizzle on the roasted veggies is a delight to the taste buds. The creamy tahini lemon sauce doesn't weigh the dish down, and it's the perfect complement to the crispness of the roasted veggies. Honestly, I don't know anyone who would turn down this dish! If you have leftovers, they're delicious mixed into a green salad the next day.

Baked Cauliflower and Broccoli

1 bunch broccoli, chopped into bite-size pieces
1 head cauliflower, chopped into bite-size pieces
2 tablespoons (30 mL) extra-virgin olive oil
½ teaspoon (2 mL) sea salt

Tahini Lemon Sauce

2 tablespoons (30 mL) tahini
1 tablespoon (15 mL) filtered water
1 tablespoon (15 mL) lemon juice
Pinch of sea salt

1. **Prepare the Baked Cauliflower and Broccoli** Preheat the oven to 350°F (180°C). Line a baking sheet with parchment paper. (You might need 2 baking sheets.)

2. Spread the broccoli and cauliflower on the prepared baking sheet. Leave a little space between the pieces, and use 2 baking sheets if necessary. Toss with olive oil to coat the vegetables and sprinkle with sea salt. Bake for 20 to 25 minutes, until golden brown and tender.

3. **Meanwhile, make the Tahini Lemon Sauce** In a small bowl, whisk together the tahini, water, lemon juice and sea salt. If the dressing is too thick, add a bit more water.

4. Transfer the roasted broccoli and cauliflower to a large serving dish and drizzle with the Tahini Lemon Sauce. Serve immediately.

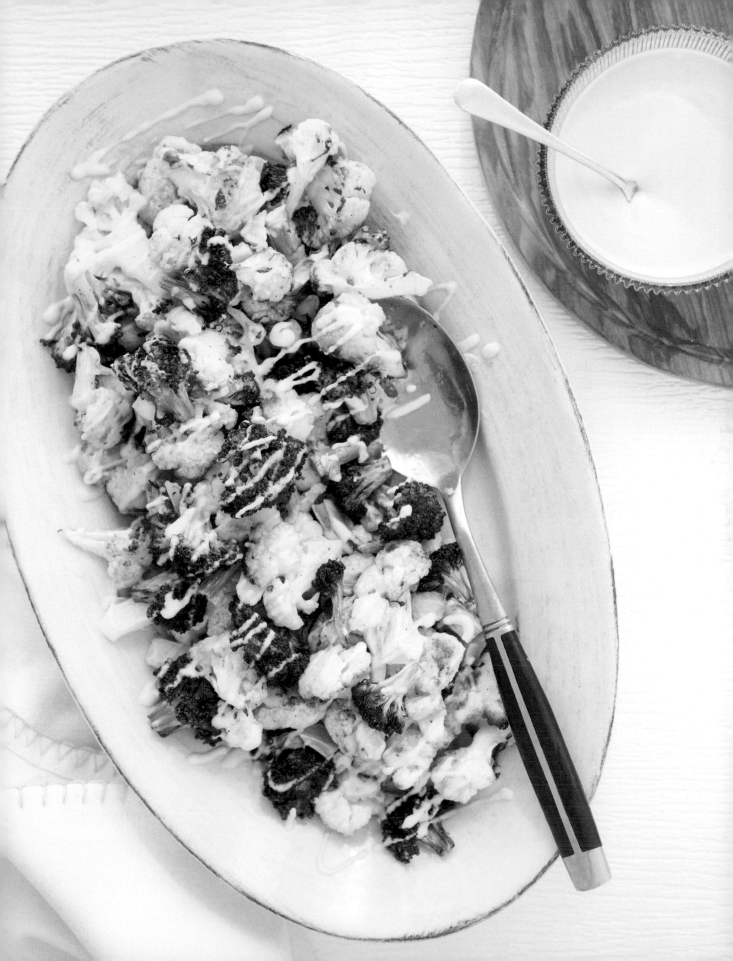

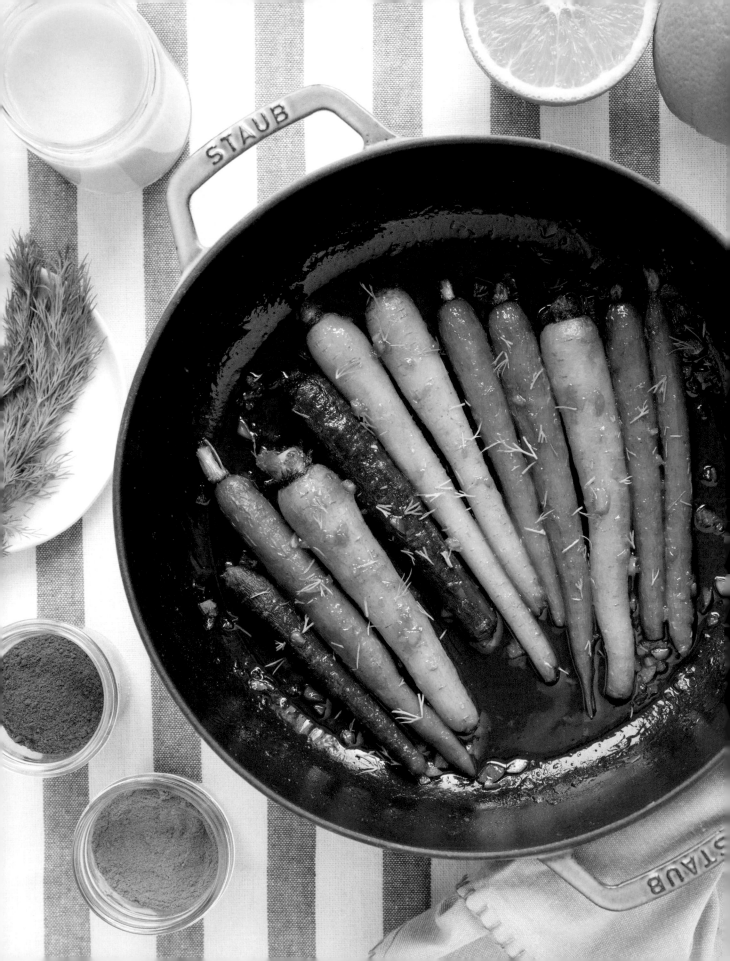

Sticky Turmeric Paprika Carrots

Gluten-free • Grain-free • Nut-free • Vegetarian

Serves 4

Typically I roast carrots because it requires very little thought. But this recipe is so incredibly tasty, I like making the extra effort for special occasions. The delicious combination of citrus, turmeric and paprika makes these sticky carrots truly memorable! Festive get-togethers aside, I love making these just for my family on chilly fall evenings.

3 heaping tablespoons (54 mL) Original Ghee (page 43), store-bought ghee or coconut oil, more as needed

4 cloves garlic, finely chopped

½ teaspoon (2 mL) ground turmeric

¼ teaspoon (1 mL) sweet paprika

Juice of 2 oranges

2 tablespoons (30 mL) real maple syrup

10 to 12 medium carrots

Pinch of sea salt

½ cup (125 mL) filtered water, as needed

1. Melt the ghee in a large frying pan over medium heat. Add the garlic and cook, stirring occasionally, for 1 minute.

2. Sprinkle the turmeric and paprika in the pan and add the orange juice and maple syrup. Stir to combine. Add the carrots, spreading them out in a single layer. Sprinkle with the sea salt. Jiggle the pan to coat the carrots with the juice mixture. Cover, reduce the heat to medium-low and simmer, stirring occasionally, for 20 minutes, or until the carrots are fork-tender. Add water as needed if the pan starts to look dry.

3. Once the carrots are cooked, remove the lid and cook, turning the carrots occasionally, for another 4 to 5 minutes, until the sauce has reduced and the carrots have begun to caramelize and are well coated with the glaze. Serve immediately.

Roasted Root Veggies

Dairy-free • Gluten-free • Grain-free • Kid-friendly • Nut-free • Vegan

Serves 6 to 8

Oh, how I adore the crispy, rich, roasted flavour of these root veggies. This dish is both comforting and fulfilling. I love making a big batch of these veggies on a Sunday afternoon to enjoy in salads all week long. They're a perfect match for my Baked Chicken with Dijon Maple Marinade (page 166) or Lamb Chops with Orange Mint Marmalade (page 200).

One way to get these veggies nice and crispy is to chop them up a few hours before roasting and leave them out on the counter, uncovered, to let the surface moisture evaporate. This helps to get those crispy outsides—and who doesn't love roasted veggies nice and crispy!

3 cups (750 mL) chopped sweet potatoes
2 cups (500 mL) chopped red beets (unpeeled if organic)
2 cups (500 mL) chopped parsnips or carrots
1 red onion, chopped
5 cloves garlic, cut in half
2 tablespoons (30 mL) extra-virgin olive oil, more for serving
2 tablespoons (30 mL) dried rosemary
½ teaspoon (2 mL) coarse sea salt
2 bunches lacinato kale, centre stems removed, roughly chopped
2 teaspoons (10 mL) balsamic vinegar
Pinch of sea salt

1. Preheat the oven to 350°F (180°C). Line a baking sheet with parchment paper.

2. In a large bowl, combine the sweet potatoes, beets, parsnips, red onion, garlic, olive oil, rosemary and coarse sea salt. Toss gently to coat.

3. Scrape the veggie mixture into a large baking dish. (If you don't have a large baking dish, use a second baking sheet lined with parchment paper. You'll just have to be careful they don't burn. Also, they will dry out more easily on a baking sheet.) Roast for 40 to 50 minutes, until the veggies are fork-tender and crisp. Remove from the oven.

4. Evenly spread the kale on the prepared baking sheet. Drizzle lightly with the balsamic vinegar and sprinkle with sea salt. Roast for 5 to 10 minutes or until crisp. Watch carefully to make sure the kale doesn't burn.

5. Combine the roasted veggies and kale in a large serving dish. Drizzle with olive oil and serve immediately.

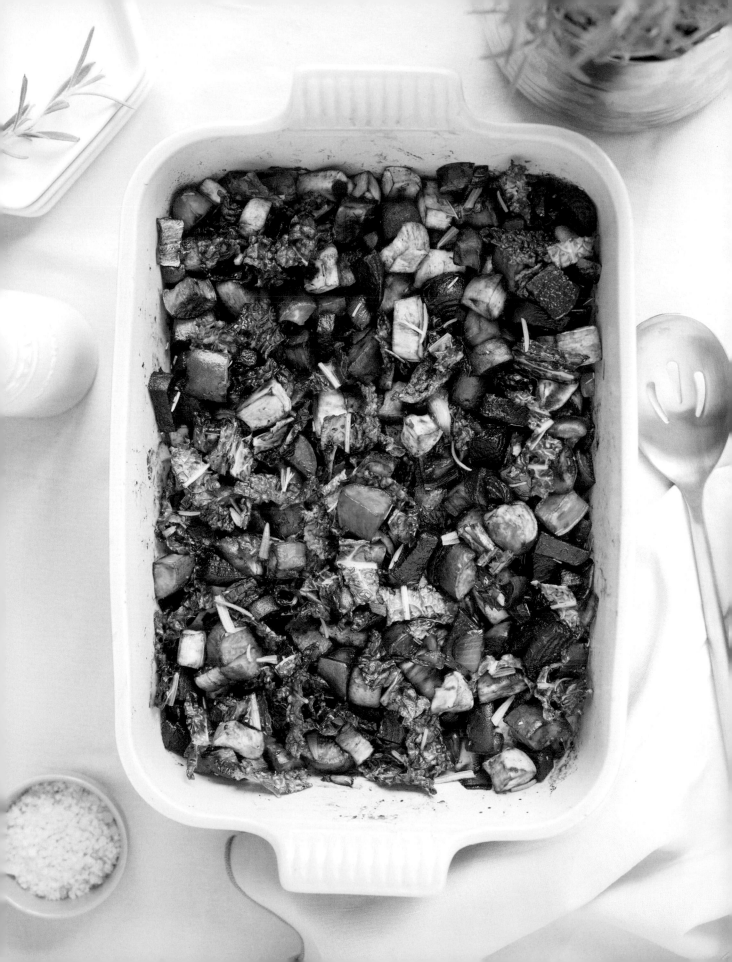

Garlicky Green Beans with Tahini Lemon Sauce

Gluten-free • Grain-free • Kid-friendly • Vegetarian

Serves 4

We discovered our love for garlicky green beans at our favourite pizzeria. Typical parents, there we were at a pizza place worrying about the lack of green foods in our daughter's diet. Which is why we ordered the garlic green beans. To our surprise, Vienna dug right in, eating them two and three at a time. Who would have thought a toddler would love garlicky green beans! Now I make them all the time for her and she still loves them.

   You can use butter in place of the ghee, but I really love ghee because it remains stable at a higher temperature. Also, if you're sensitive to dairy protein, ghee is an excellent choice because there is no (or very little) milk protein present. And besides, it tastes delicious! These green beans go really well with my Quinoa-Stuffed Spaghetti Squash (page 195). If you're feeling like pizza, then try them alongside any of the Super-Quick Tortilla Pizzas (page175).

Garlicky Green Beans

1 tablespoon (15 mL) Original Ghee (page 43), store-bought ghee or extra-virgin olive oil
4 cloves garlic, chopped
3 cups (750 mL) green beans, trimmed
¼ cup (60 mL) chopped raw or roasted almonds
¼ cup (60 mL) pomegranate seeds
3 tablespoons (45 mL) nutritional yeast

Tahini Lemon Sauce

2 tablespoons (30 mL) tahini
1 tablespoon (15 mL) filtered water
1 tablespoon (15 mL) lemon juice
Pinch of sea salt

1. **Make the Garlicky Green Beans** Melt the Original Ghee in a large frying pan over medium heat. Add the garlic and cook, stirring occasionally, for 2 minutes, until fragrant. Add a splash of water if the pan gets too hot to prevent the garlic from burning. Add the green beans and cook, stirring occasionally, for 10 to 15 minutes, until the beans are fork-tender but not soggy.

2. **Meanwhile, make the Tahini Lemon Sauce** In a small bowl, whisk together the tahini, water, lemon juice and sea salt. If the dressing is too thick, add a bit more water.

3. Transfer the green beans to a bowl or plate. Drizzle with the Tahini Lemon Sauce and garnish with the almonds, pomegranate seeds and nutritional yeast. Serve immediately.

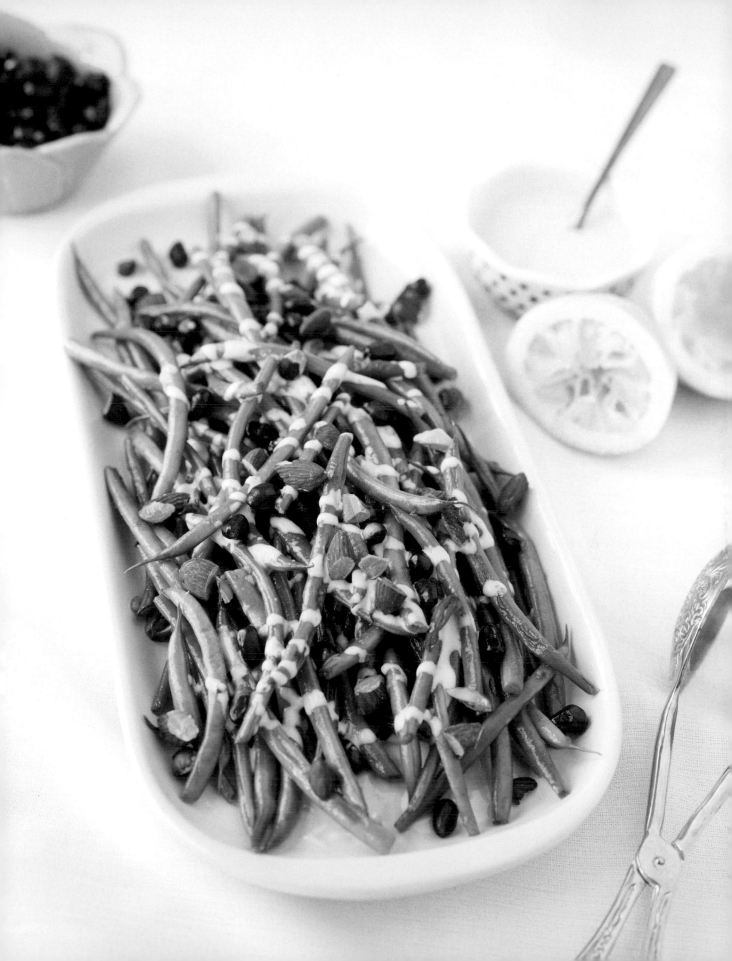

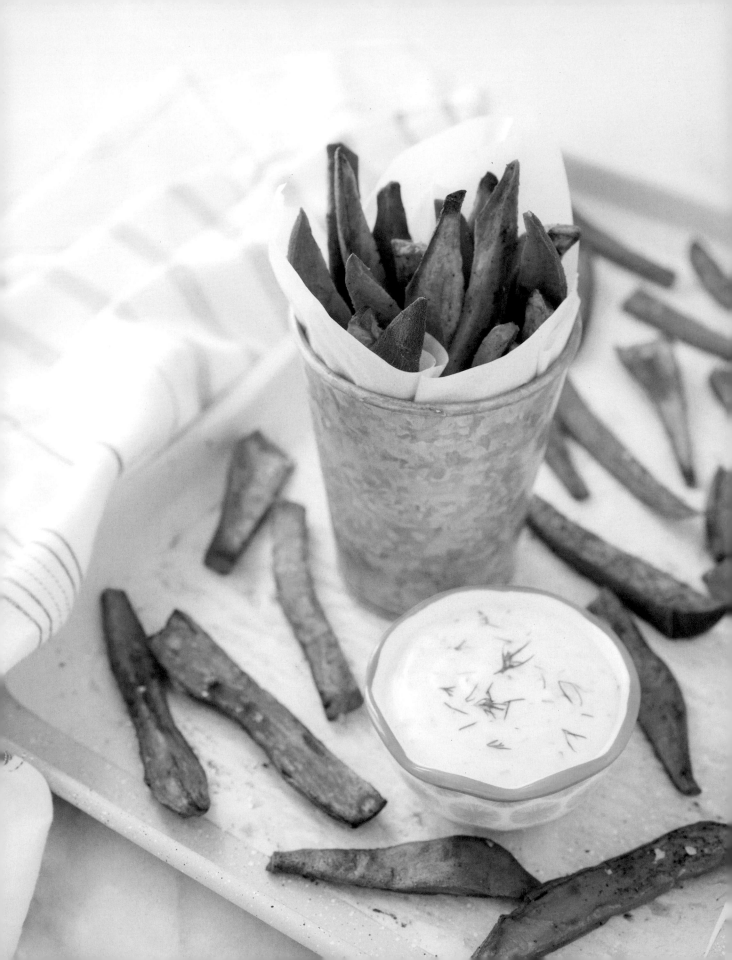

Curry Sweet Potato Wedges with Yogurt Dill Dip

Gluten-free · Grain-free · Kid-friendly · Nut-free · Vegetarian

Serves 4 to 6

I eat my weight in sweet potatoes every winter, and then some! I love sweet potato wedges, and they are always a hit at family dinners. If it's just me and my hubs, Walker, I will make them nice and crispy. If our daughter, Vienna, is eating them too, I cook them until they're soft but skip cranking the temperature up to make them crispy on the outside.

You won't need any ketchup with these wedges because they are super delicious with this healthy yogurt dip. These wedges are a perfect match with my Crispy Chicken Fingers with Barbecue Sauce (page 176).

Yogurt Dill Dip

½ cup (125 mL) unsweetened plain
　full-fat yogurt or coconut yogurt
Juice of 1 lime
1 clove garlic, minced
1 tablespoon (15 mL) chopped fresh dill

Curry Sweet Potato Wedges

4 sweet potatoes, sliced into wedges
2 tablespoons (30 mL) extra-virgin olive oil
½ teaspoon (2 mL) coarse sea salt
½ teaspoon (2 mL) curry powder
¼ teaspoon (1 mL) cayenne pepper
　(optional)

1. **Make the Yogurt Dill Dip** In a small bowl, whisk together the yogurt, lime juice, garlic and dill. Set aside.

2. **Prepare the Curry Sweet Potato Wedges** Preheat the oven to 375°F (190°C). Line a baking sheet with parchment paper.

3. Place the potato wedges in a large bowl and drizzle with the olive oil. Sprinkle with sea salt, curry powder and cayenne, if using. Toss to coat the wedges. Spread the wedges evenly on the prepared baking sheet. Bake for 25 to 30 minutes, until fork-tender. If you want crispy wedges, increase the heat to 400°F (200°C) for the last 5 minutes of cooking. Be careful not to burn them. Serve hot with the Yogurt Dill Dip on the side.

Mushroom, Asparagus and Feta Tartines

Nut-free • Vegetarian

Makes 4 tartines

This tartine is bursting with so much flavour, honestly it makes my mouth water when I'm preparing it. It's welcome any time of day, as an appetizer before dinner, a side to go with soup like my Broccoli and Leek Soup with Herbaceous Croutons (page 143) or for breakfast with a poached egg on top.

You can toast the sourdough bread in a toaster or pop the slices on a baking sheet, drizzle with olive oil and bake at 425°F (220°C) until golden and a little crispy. Just be careful not to burn the bread. If you're making this as an appetizer for a larger group, just cut each slice of bread smaller and you'll get more than four tartines.

2 tablespoons (30 mL) extra-virgin olive oil

¼ cup (60 mL) finely chopped white onion

2 cloves garlic, finely chopped

8 ounces (225 g) cremini mushrooms, sliced

2 teaspoons (10 mL) real maple syrup

1 teaspoon (5 mL) gluten-free tamari

1 teaspoon (5 mL) dried thyme

¼ teaspoon (1 mL) dried oregano

1 cup (250 mL) chopped trimmed asparagus

4 slices of sourdough bread (½ inch/1 cm thick), toasted or grilled

¼ cup (60 mL) crumbled feta cheese

Pepper

1. In a large frying pan, heat the olive oil over medium heat. Add the onion and garlic and cook, stirring occasionally, until the onions are soft and transparent, about 4 minutes. Add the mushrooms and cook for 5 more minutes.

2. Stir in the maple syrup, tamari, thyme, oregano and asparagus. Cook for 5 minutes, or until the asparagus is fork-tender. If the pan is getting dry, add a splash of water.

3. To assemble, evenly divide the mushroom mixture between the slices of toasted sourdough bread. Top with feta and sprinkle with pepper to taste. Serve immediately.

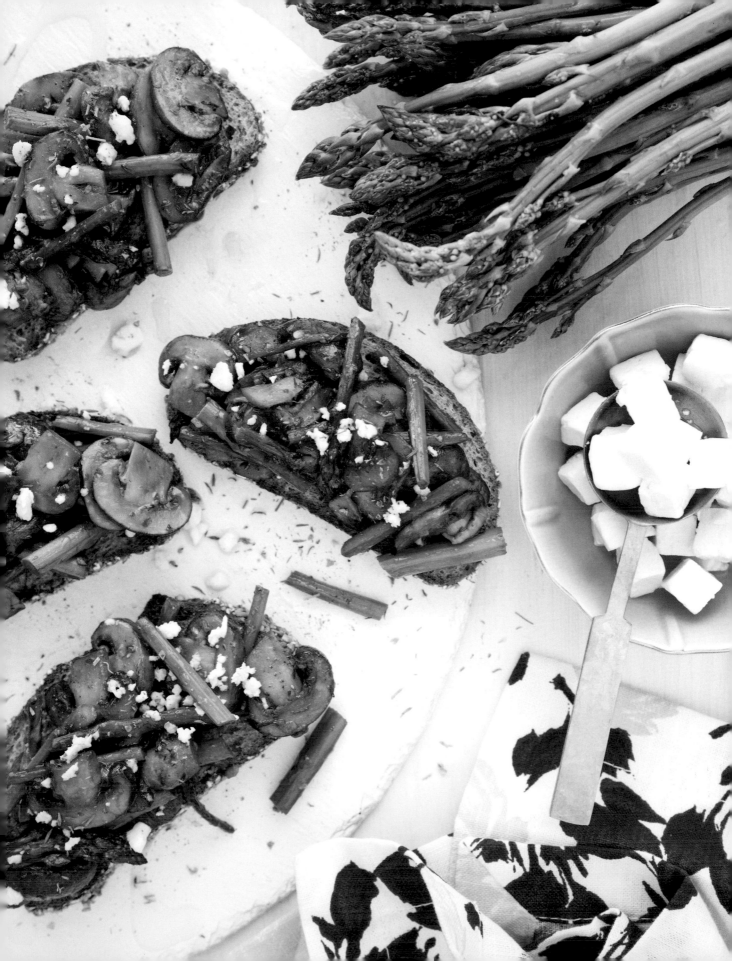

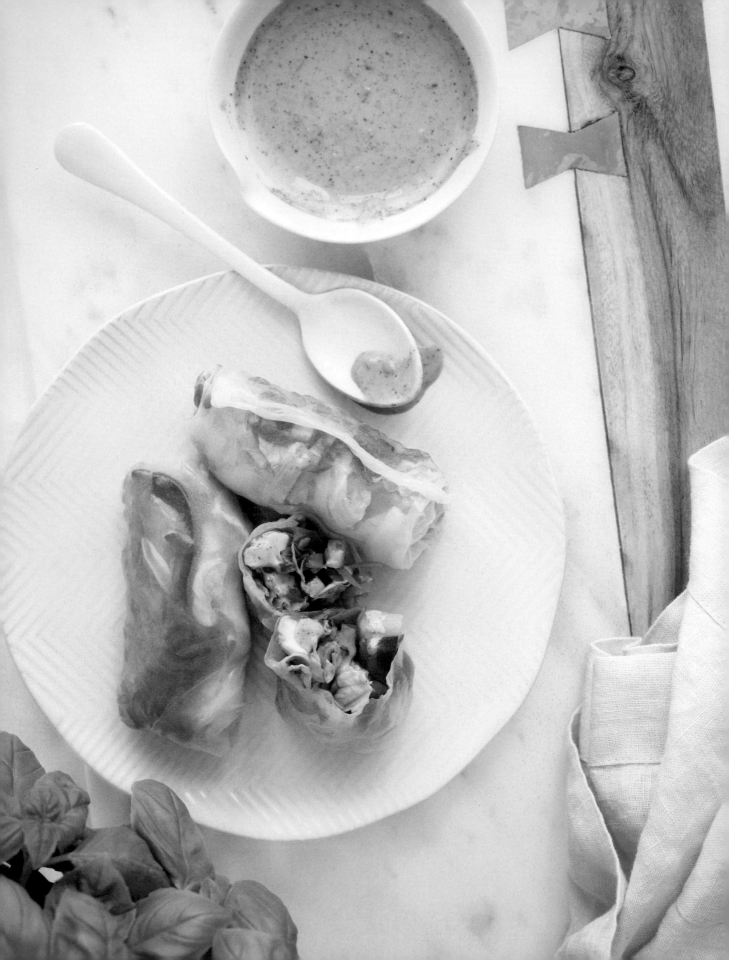

Veggie Rolls with Spicy Almond Sauce

Dairy-free • Gluten-free • Grain-free • Kid-friendly • Vegan

Makes 8 veggie rolls

An easy snack or appetizer, these rice-paper wraps are super fun to make and are always a hit when entertaining! I let my leftovers dictate what I will stuff in them and often use whatever produce is in my fridge before it goes bad.

Rice-paper wrappers can be found at health food stores, the Asian section of the grocery store or specialty food stores. If you can't find them locally, you'll be able to find them online. They're sticky when wet, but once you get the hang of assembling the first one, you'll be a pro.

Spicy Almond Sauce

¼ cup (60 mL) tahini
¼ cup (60 mL) natural almond butter
1 tablespoon (15 mL) gluten-free tamari
1 teaspoon (5 mL) grated fresh ginger
1 clove garlic, minced
Juice of 1 lime
½ teaspoon (2 mL) cayenne pepper
4 to 6 tablespoons (60 to 90 mL) filtered
  water, for desired consistency

Rice-Paper Veggie Rolls

1 cup (250 mL) boiling water,
  for soaking the wrappers
8 rice-paper wrappers
4 carrots, grated
1 cup (250 mL) shredded romaine lettuce
2 ripe mangos, peeled and thinly sliced
1 sweet red pepper, cut into matchsticks
2 ripe avocados, pitted, peeled and sliced
8 fresh basil leaves
8 fresh mint leaves

1. **Make the Spicy Almond Sauce** In a small bowl, whisk together the tahini, almond butter, tamari, ginger, garlic, lime juice and cayenne. Whisk in enough water to reach the consistency you like.

2. **Assemble the Rice-Paper Veggie Rolls** Pour the boiling water into a round cake pan or pie pan and let cool for 3 minutes. Working with one rice-paper wrapper at a time, immerse it in the hot water until softened, about 30 seconds. Use both hands to carefully remove the softened wrapper and place it on a work surface. In the centre of the wrapper, quickly arrange a small amount of the carrots, some lettuce, 1 or 2 slices of mango, red pepper, avocado, and 1 leaf each of basil and mint.

3. To roll up the wrapper, first fold the bottom and top edges over the filling, then fold in one side toward the centre and continue rolling the filled wrapper until closed and snug. Repeat filling and rolling the remaining veggie rolls. If not serving right away, store in the fridge until ready to eat.

4. Serve with the Spicy Almond Sauce on the side.

Zucchini Fritters

Gluten-free • Kid-friendly • Vegetarian

Makes about 10 fritters

When summer squash is in season, you see yellow and green zucchini at every farmers' market in town. They aren't hard to grow, but the larger the zucchini, the tougher in texture it can be, so big doesn't necessarily mean better. I look for medium-size zucchini for the best flavour and texture for these mouth-watering fritters.

Zucchini is one of those foods you don't really think of as being a health superstar like kale or broccoli, but it is an amazing source of pectin, a fibre that supports gut and cardiovascular health. The cool thing about this fibre is that it prevents cholesterol from being reabsorbed back into the body! If you have zucchini left over after making these fritters, then try my Zucchini Noodles with Turkey Meatballs (page 196) or Zucchini Blueberry Loaf (page 22).

2 cups (500 mL) grated zucchini

1 large egg

1 small red onion, finely chopped

½ cup (125 mL) quinoa flour or almond flour (almond meal)

½ cup (125 mL) grated goat cheddar cheese, Parmesan cheese or non-dairy cheese

½ cup (125 mL) loosely packed chopped fresh basil

2 teaspoons (10 mL) dried rosemary

1 teaspoon (5 mL) garlic powder (or 2 cloves garlic, minced)

Pinch each of sea salt and pepper

2 tablespoons (30 mL) coconut oil, for frying

1. Preheat the oven to 350°F (180°C). Line a baking sheet with parchment paper.

2. Place the grated zucchini in a fine-mesh strainer or nut milk bag and press or wring out excess water. Don't skip this step or your fritters will be too wet.

3. In a large bowl, whisk the egg, then whisk in the zucchini, red onion, quinoa flour, cheese, basil, rosemary, garlic powder, sea salt and pepper. Form into about 10 patties, each 3 to 4 inches (8 to 10 cm) round.

4. Melt the coconut oil in a large frying pan over medium heat. Working in batches, cook the fritters for 5 minutes, until the bottom starts to turn golden brown. Flip and cook for another 5 minutes, until golden brown. Be careful not to let the fritters burn—you just want to sear the outside.

5. Place the fritters as they're fried on the prepared baking sheet. When all the fritters are fried, bake for 20 to 25 minutes, until golden.

6. Enjoy immediately or store in an airtight container in the fridge for up to 5 days. Reheat in the oven at 350°F (180°C) for 10 minutes.

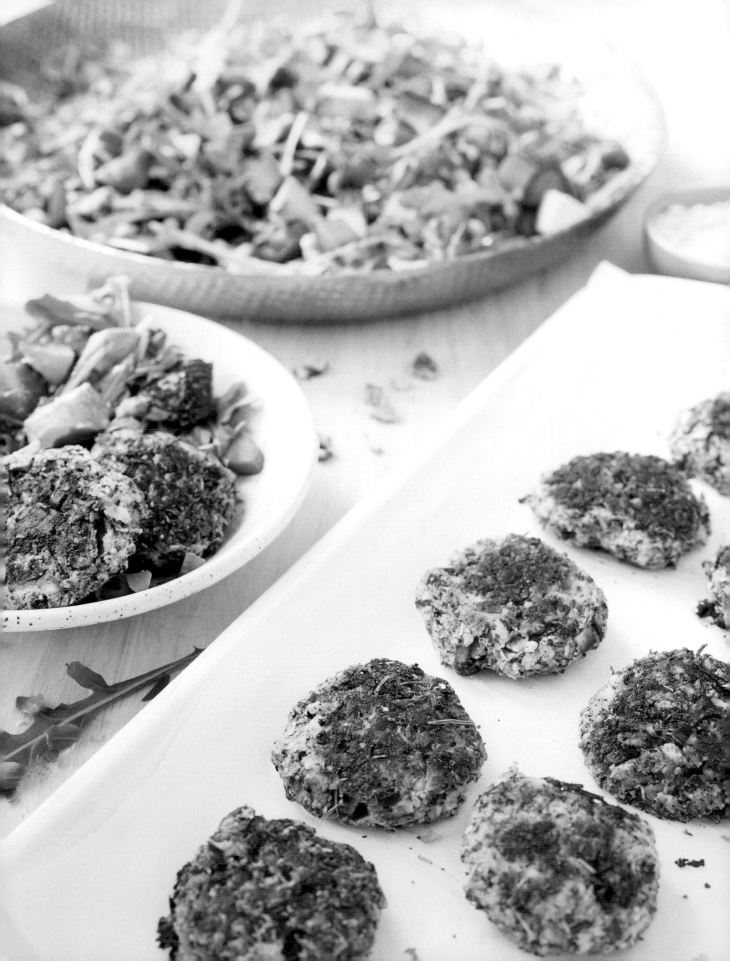

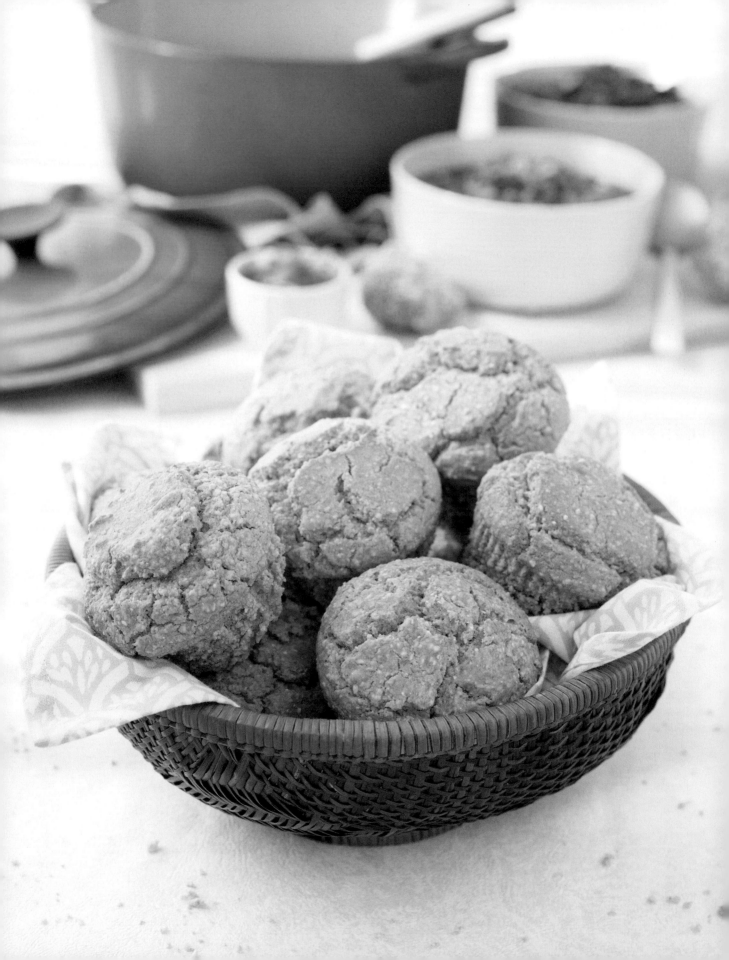

Spicy Cornbread Muffins

Dairy-free • Gluten-free • Kid-friendly • Vegetarian

Makes 24 muffins

Cornbread is to chili or soup what ice cream is to apple pie! I always make a batch of these cornbread muffins when I'm having a hot one-pot meal like my Slow Cooker Spicy Turkey Chili (page 161) or Roasted Pear and Parsnip Soup (page 148). They are pretty dense and filling, so you don't have to worry about eating the whole batch—you'll be full after one!

If you're making these for kids who aren't crazy about spicy, you can simply omit the jalapeño peppers. They are just as delicious! If you want them a little sweeter, you can add cinnamon and increase the coconut sugar by a couple of tablespoons.

1½ cups (375 mL) brown rice flour
1½ cups (375 mL) cornmeal
¼ cup (60 mL) coconut sugar
2 teaspoons (10 mL) baking powder
1 teaspoon (5 mL) baking soda
1 teaspoon (5 mL) sea salt
2 eggs
1½ cups (375 mL) unsweetened almond milk
6 tablespoons (90 mL) extra-virgin olive oil
2 tablespoons (30 mL) real maple syrup
2 jalapeño peppers, seeded and finely chopped (optional)

1. Position the oven racks in the top third and lower third of the oven and preheat the oven to 350°F (180°C). Line 2 muffin tins with paper liners.

2. In a large bowl, whisk together the brown rice flour, cornmeal, coconut sugar, baking powder, baking soda and sea salt.

3. In a medium bowl, whisk the eggs, then whisk in the almond milk, olive oil and maple syrup. Add the wet mixture to the dry mixture and stir just until combined. Fold in the jalapeños, if using.

4. Fill the muffin cups about three-quarters full. Bake, rotating the muffin tins top to bottom and front to back halfway through, for 15 to 20 minutes, until the muffins are golden brown on top and a fork inserted in the centre of a muffin comes out clean.

5. Transfer the muffins to a rack and let cool completely. Store in an airtight container in the fridge for up to 5 days or in the freezer for up to 3 months.

Za'atar Socca

Dairy-free • Gluten-free • Grain-free • Kid-friendly • Nut-free • Vegan

Serves 4

I first tasted za'atar at a Middle Eastern restaurant, and when I saw it at my local health food store a few weeks later, I bought some to experiment with at home. Za'atar is a blend of aromatic dried herbs—often thyme, oregano and marjoram—plus sumac and sesame seeds. Depending on who you ask, it has different pronunciations, but I say "zah-tar." It's very simple to make your own za'atar blend, but it's also convenient to buy it already blended. Za'atar jazzes up any recipe, whether it's a dip, barbecued chicken or this socca, making it a welcome addition to the spice cupboard.

Socca is a flatbread made with chickpea flour, and za'atar takes this socca to the next level of deliciousness. This socca is perfect with soup, such as my Creamy Cremini Mushroom Soup (page 144) or Roasted Red Pepper Soup (page 148).

1 cup (250 mL) chickpea flour
1 cup (250 mL) filtered water
2 tablespoons (30 mL) extra-virgin
   olive oil, more for serving
2 cloves garlic, minced
1 tablespoon (15 mL) za'atar
½ teaspoon (2 mL) sea salt
Pinch of freshly ground black pepper
Pinch of red chili flakes (optional)

1. Preheat the oven to 400°F (200°C). Grease an 8-inch (20 cm) round baking pan or cast-iron frying pan.

2. In a large bowl, whisk together the chickpea flour, water, oil and garlic. Pour the mixture into the baking pan and sprinkle with za'atar, sea salt, pepper and chili flakes, if using.

3. Bake for 22 minutes, or until the socca is crisp around the edges and golden brown. I like to put the oven on broil for a few minutes at the end to get the socca nice and brown.

4. The socca is best served hot but can be stored in an airtight container in the fridge for up to 1 week. Reheat in the oven or toaster. Drizzle with olive oil just before serving.

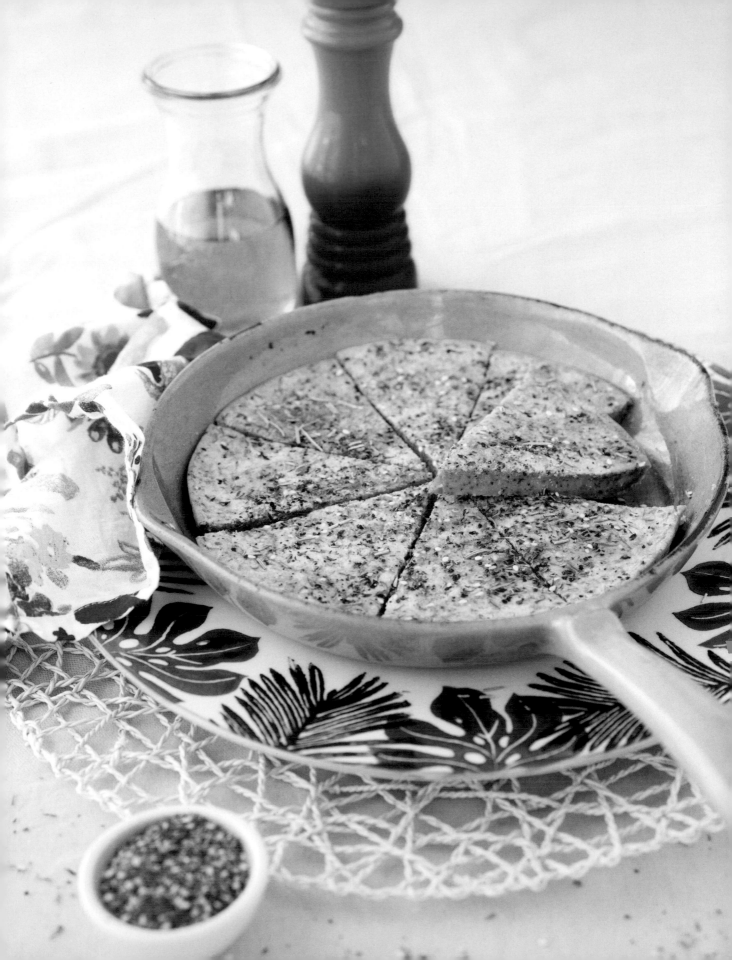

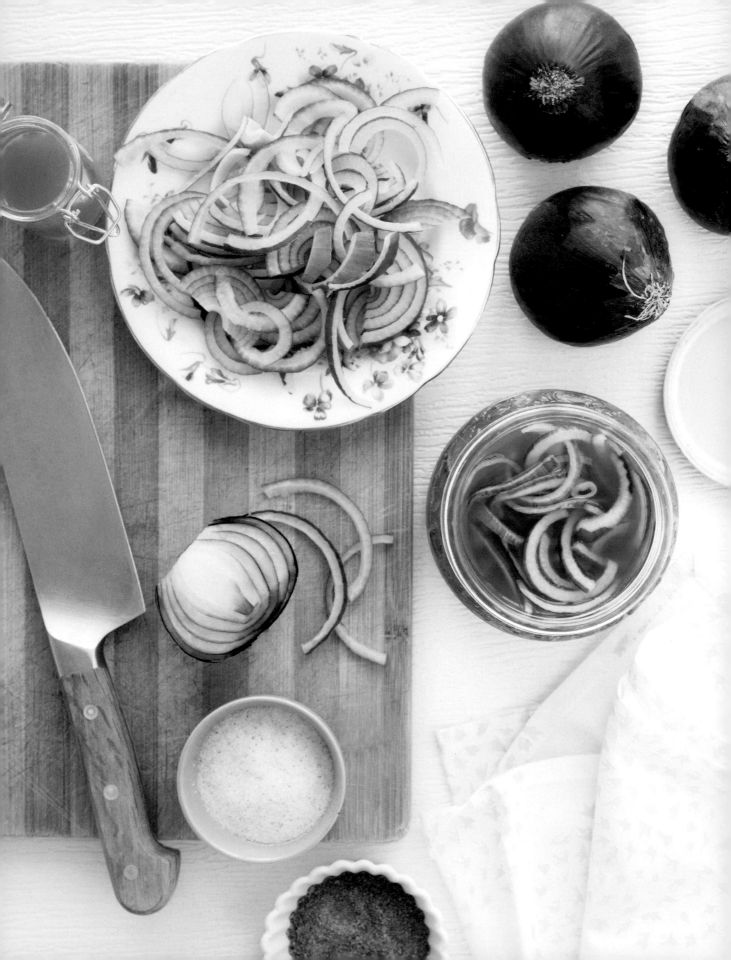

Quick Pickled Onions

Dairy-free · Gluten-free · Grain-free · Nut-free · Vegan

Makes 1 to 1½ cups (250 to 375 mL)

These pickled onions go in just about every salad, sandwich and wrap I make because they add that extra punch of flavour. I also like putting them on a charcuterie board when entertaining. It's really a no-brainer to always have these stocked in my fridge because they are so easy to make. This pickling method works for just about any veggie and it works for pickled eggs, too.

1 medium red onion, thinly sliced
1 cup (250 mL) filtered water, at room temperature
½ cup (125 mL) apple cider vinegar
1 tablespoon (15 mL) coconut sugar
1 teaspoon (5 mL) fine sea salt

1. Place the red onion in a large mason jar.

2. In a small bowl, whisk together the water, apple cider vinegar, coconut sugar and sea salt until the sugar and salt are dissolved. Pour over the sliced onions. Screw the lid on tight and give it a good shake. Store in the fridge for up to 2 weeks.

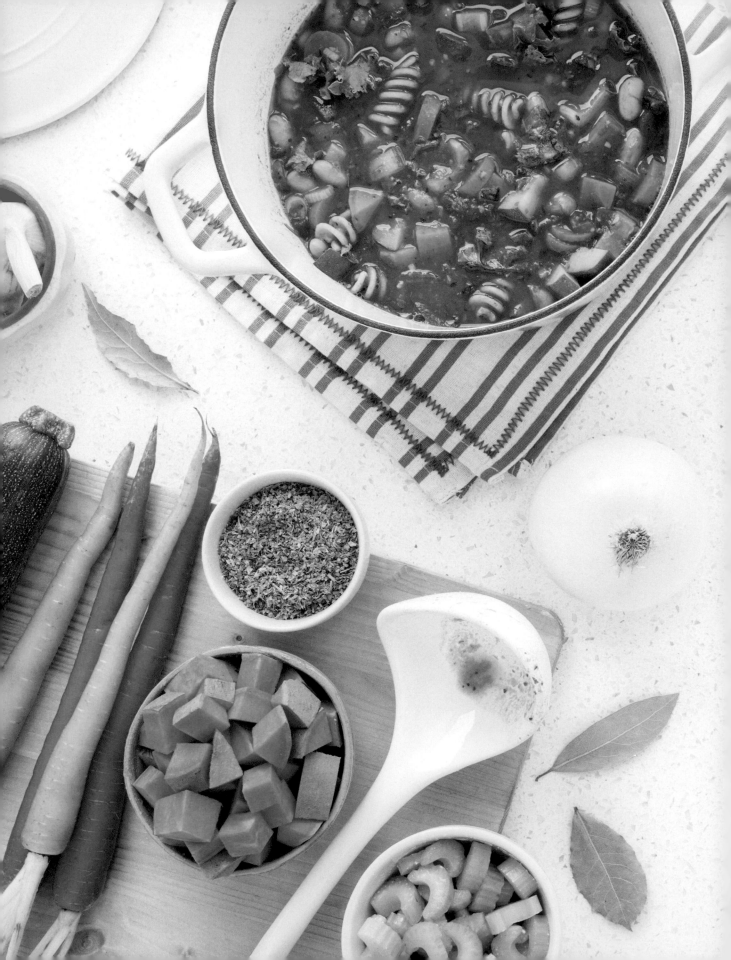

Soups and One-Pot Meals

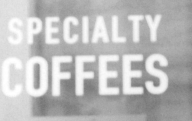SPECIALTY
COFFEES

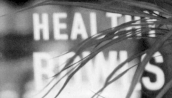HEALTHY
BOWLS

SOUPS AND ONE-POT MEALS

One-pot meals are all about simplicity. Sure, the finished dish may be rich and complex, but the prep is meant to be as easy as "toss everything in and go!" You will probably find that you already have most of the non-perishable ingredients on hand and only need to buy a few fresh items to make a delicious, satisfying meal. In this chapter I share an amazing blend of old family favourites and new recipes that are great for batch cooking and nourishing to the core. My Slow Cooker Spicy Turkey Chili (page 161) is perfect for the deep winter chill or if you're hosting a big group for dinner and you want a meal that you can make ahead.

I love making a batch of soup on a Sunday afternoon so I have lunch already done for a few days during the work week. This chapter is full of delicious and hearty soups that you can enjoy all year long, like Mamabea's Seafood Soup (page 151), which is packed with flavour and protein, making it an entire meal on its own, or my Butternut Squash Lentil Soup (page 152), which can also be easily blended into a purée for little ones.

Remember that one-pot meals and soups aren't just for the cooler months either. My Chilled Zucchini Avocado Basil Soup (page 139) is super refreshing in the summer, and my Roasted Red Pepper Soup (page 148) is welcome any time of the year.

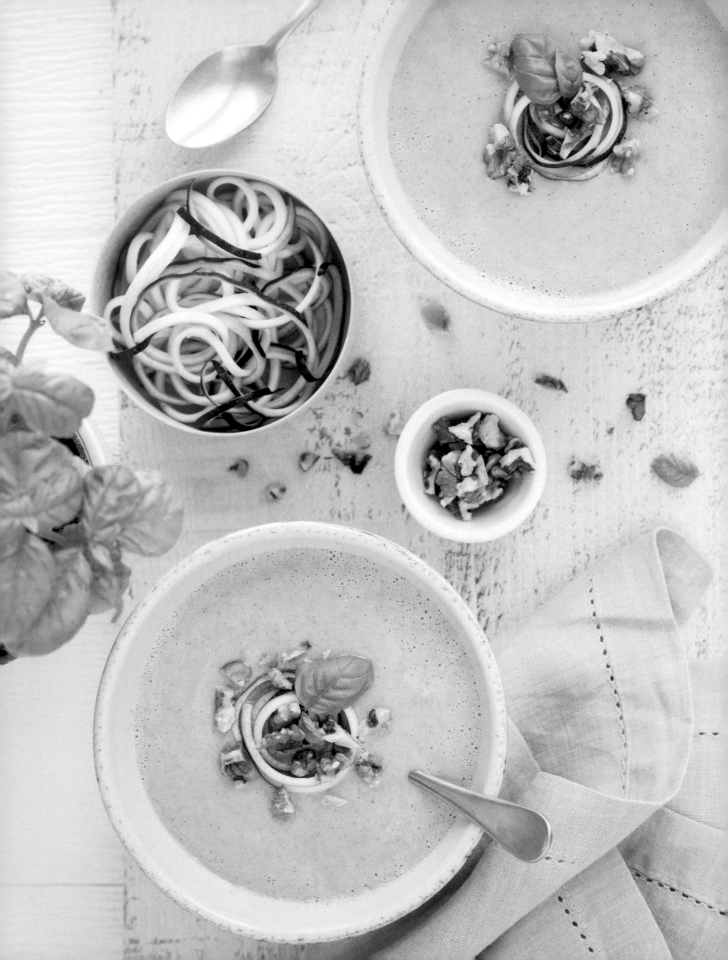

Chilled Zucchini Avocado Basil Soup

Dairy-free · Gluten-free · Grain-free · Kid-friendly · Vegan

Serves 4

I stick to a list when shopping at the grocery store, but when I go to a farmers' market, I am a little more reckless. I tend to shop based on what is inspiring me—otherwise known as shopping on impulse. I'm such a sucker when a farmer tells me they picked something just a few hours ago. That's definitely a great sales pitch for me, because the more recently it was picked, the richer in vitamins it will be.

I love making this soup when I've bought too many zucchini at the market and need to make good use of them before they go bad. This dairy-free soup is still nice and creamy because avocados provide a wonderful richness. It goes well with my Summer Salad with Halloumi (page 96). If you still have zucchini hanging around after making this soup, then definitely try my Zucchini Blueberry Loaf (page 22) or Zucchini Fritters (page 126).

2 tablespoons (30 mL) extra-virgin olive oil

1 small white onion, chopped

1 clove garlic, chopped

4 zucchini, chopped

Juice of 1 lemon

1 ripe avocado, pitted, peeled and roughly chopped

1 cup (250 mL) loosely packed fresh basil leaves

2 to 3 cups (500 to 750 mL) vegetable stock, divided

2 tablespoons (30 mL) chopped raw walnuts, for garnish

1. Heat the olive oil in a medium frying pan over medium heat. Add the onion and garlic and cook, stirring occasionally, until the onions are soft and translucent, about 4 minutes. Add the zucchini and continue cooking for 5 to 7 minutes, until the zucchini starts to soften.

2. Transfer the zucchini mixture to a high-speed blender. Add the lemon juice, avocado, basil and 2 cups (500 mL) of the vegetable stock. Blend until smooth. Add up to 1 cup (250 mL) stock for a thinner consistency.

3. Refrigerate for at least 4 hours. Serve chilled, garnished with walnuts. Store in an airtight container in the fridge for up to 1 week.

Turmeric Butternut Squash Soup

Dairy-free • Gluten-free • Grain-free • Kid-friendly • Nut-free • Vegan

Serves 4 to 6

Butternut squash is a foolproof ingredient. Even if you added no other ingredients and just puréed the roasted squash, it would taste amazing. This was one of the first soups that I introduced to my daughter, Vienna, after she was already sold on turmeric from my Turmeric Ginger Latte (page 69).

   You can use 2-inch (5 cm) pieces of fresh turmeric and ginger for this recipe. I used ground turmeric because it's easier to find than fresh. Occasionally I add a can of full-fat coconut milk for added richness, but the butternut squash gets nice and creamy all on its own.

3 to 4 cups (750 mL to 1 L) peeled and
   cubed butternut squash (about 1 large)
2 tablespoons (30 mL) + ½ teaspoon
   (2 mL) extra-virgin olive oil, divided
4 to 6 cups (1 L to 1.5 L) vegetable stock,
   divided
2 white onions (or 6 shallots), chopped
Juice of ½ lemon
1 teaspoon (5 mL) ground turmeric
½ teaspoon (2 mL) ground ginger
4 lacinato kale leaves, centre stems
   removed, chopped
Pinch of sea salt
¼ cup (60 mL) Roasted Chickpeas
   (page 107), for garnish

1. Preheat the oven to 350°F (180°C). Line 2 baking sheets with parchment paper.

2. Spread the butternut squash cubes evenly on one baking sheet and drizzle with 1 tablespoon (15 mL) of the olive oil. Bake for 30 to 35 minutes, until fork-tender. Let cool for 10 minutes. Leave the oven on to cook the kale chips.

3. Meanwhile, heat the vegetable stock in a large pot over medium heat. Reduce the heat and keep warm.

4. Heat 1 tablespoon (15 mL) olive oil in a medium frying pan over medium heat. Add the onions and cook, stirring occasionally, until soft and translucent, about 5 minutes.

5. In a high-speed blender or food processor, combine the squash, onions, 4 (1 L) cups of the vegetable stock, lemon juice, turmeric and ginger. Blend until smooth. Add up to 2 cups (500 mL) stock for a thinner consistency, if needed. Transfer the soup to the large pot and keep warm over low heat until ready to serve.

6. To make the kale chips, spread the kale evenly on the other prepared baking sheet. Drizzle with the remaining ½ teaspoon (2 mL) olive oil and sprinkle with sea salt. Bake for 8 minutes, or until the kale is crispy. Be careful not to burn the chips.

7. Serve the soup hot, garnished with kale chips and Roasted Chickpeas. Store, without the kale and chickpeas, in an airtight container in the fridge for up to 5 days or in a mason jar in the freezer for up to 3 months.

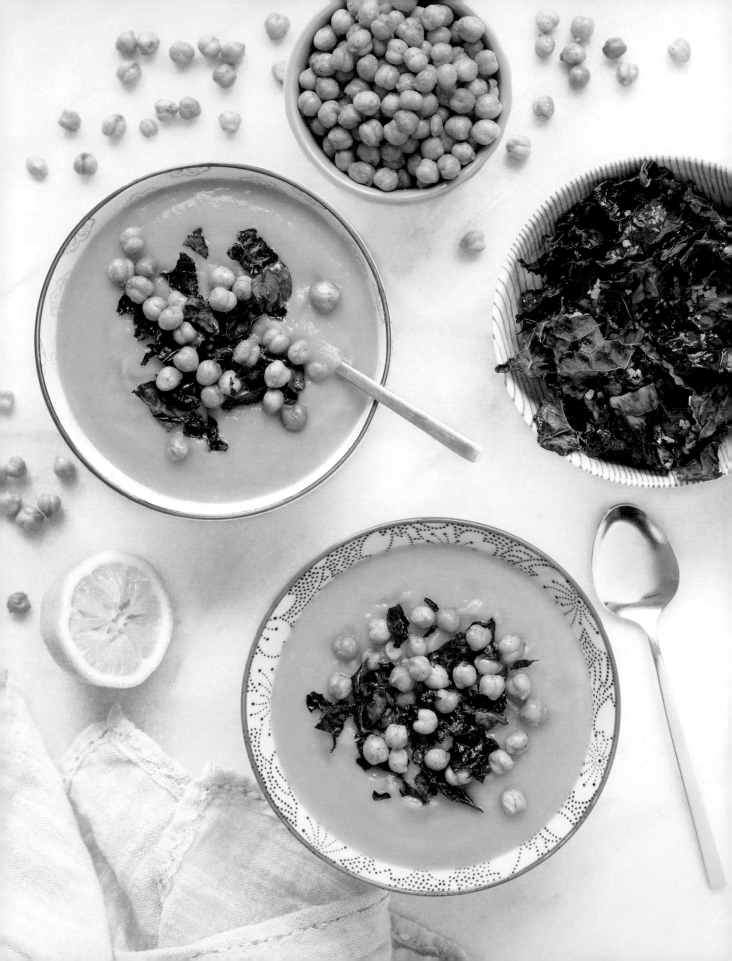

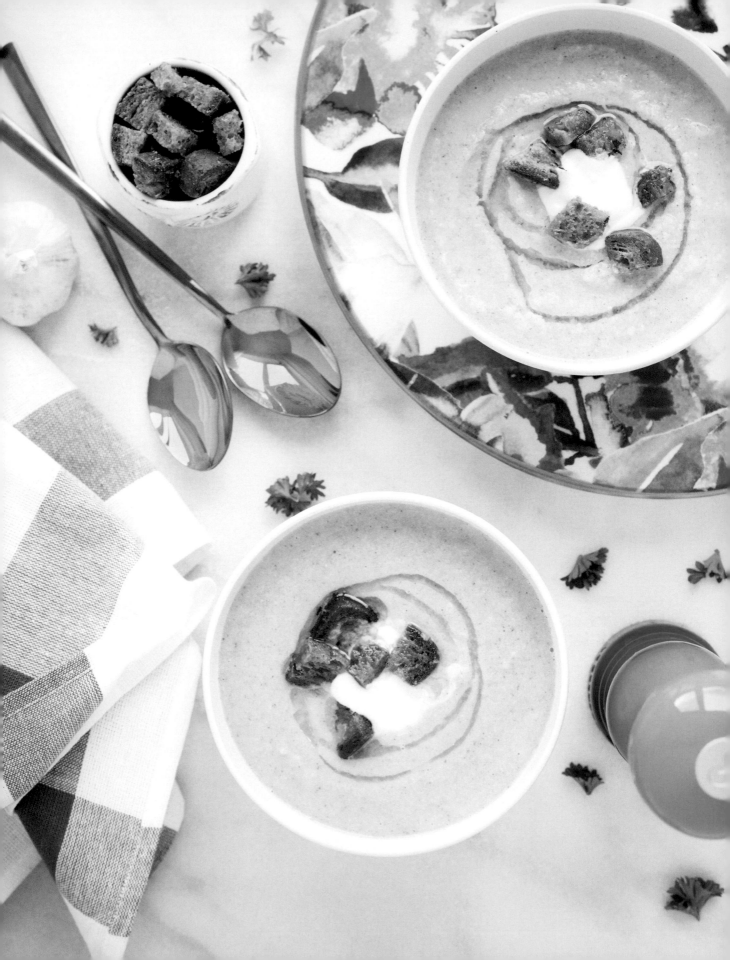

Broccoli and Leek Soup with Herbaceous Croutons

Dairy-free • Gluten-free • Nut-free • Vegan

Serves 6

With crusty, herby gluten-free croutons and a dollop of full-fat yogurt on top, this healthy and easy soup goes well with my Mushroom, Asparagus and Feta Tartines (page 122) for a fulfilling but light meal. I'm a huge fan of leeks and use them all the time when they are in season, which is often, because they have a long growing season. Leeks make pretty much any soup darn tasty, in my opinion. They have a very mild onion-like taste without taking over the flavour of this soup.

Broccoli makes this soup a winner when you consider the array of health benefits it possesses. I enjoy this soup both chilled and warm. If you like it creamier, add half a 14-ounce (400 mL) can of full-fat coconut milk.

Herbaceous Croutons

4 pieces of day-old gluten-free bread, cut into bite-size pieces
2 tablespoons (30 mL) extra-virgin olive oil
1 teaspoon (5 mL) dried rosemary
½ teaspoon (2 mL) dried thyme
½ teaspoon (2 mL) dried basil
1 teaspoon (5 mL) nutritional yeast (optional)

Broccoli and Leek Soup

2 tablespoons (30 mL) extra-virgin olive oil
2 leeks (white and light green parts only), cut in half lengthwise and thinly sliced
6 cups (1.5 L) broccoli florets
3 cups (750 mL) vegetable stock
Juice of 1 lemon
Sea salt
Plain coconut yogurt, for serving (optional)

1. **Make the Herbaceous Croutons** Preheat the oven to 350°F (180°C). Line a baking sheet with parchment paper.

2. Place the bread pieces in a large bowl and drizzle with olive oil. Sprinkle with the rosemary, thyme and basil. Toss to coat, then spread evenly on the prepared baking sheet. Bake for 10 minutes, or until golden and crispy. Remove from the oven and sprinkle with nutritional yeast, if using. Set aside until ready to use. The croutons can be stored in an airtight container at room temperature for up to 5 days.

3. **Make the Broccoli and Leek Soup** In a large pot, heat the olive oil over medium heat. Add the leeks and cook, stirring occasionally, until tender and fragrant, 4 to 5 minutes. Stir in the broccoli and cook for 5 more minutes. Add the vegetable stock and cook until the broccoli is fork-tender (not mushy). Remove from the heat and let cool for 10 minutes.

4. Transfer the broccoli mixture to a high-speed blender or food processor. Add the lemon juice and sea salt to taste. Blend until smooth. If not serving right away, return the soup to the pot and keep warm over low heat.

5. Serve the soup hot, topped with Herbaceous Croutons and a dollop of coconut yogurt, if using. Store, without the croutons and yogurt, in an airtight container in the fridge for up to 5 days or in a mason jar in the freezer for up to 3 months.

Creamy Cremini Mushroom Soup

Gluten-free · Grain-free · Nut-free · Vegetarian

Serves 4 to 6

Early in the autumn, mushrooms are calling my name. Mushrooms have such a magical way of becoming creamy when cooked and blended to perfection, people will never believe there's no cream in this soup! The earthiness of the mushrooms combined with thyme, tarragon and parsley makes this soup a memorable one.

If you can't find cremini mushrooms you can use white button mushrooms instead, although they don't taste quite as earthy. Even though the chanterelles are optional, I highly recommend using them. The meatiness of the chanterelles combined with the creaminess of the soup is pure bliss on every level. Enjoy this with some Za'atar Socca (page 130).

2 tablespoons (30 mL) coconut oil

8 ounces (225 g) cremini mushrooms, chopped

1 large white onion, chopped

2 cloves garlic, chopped

4 teaspoons (20 mL) dried tarragon

2 teaspoons (10 mL) dried parsley

1 teaspoon (5 mL) dried thyme

4 cups (1 L) vegetable stock

2 tablespoons (30 mL) Italian-Seasoned Ghee (page 44) or store-bought ghee

1 package (1.4 to 1.7 ounces/40 to 50 g) dried chanterelle mushrooms (optional)

4 teaspoons (20 mL) crumbled goat cheese, for serving

1 teaspoon (5 mL) extra-virgin olive oil, for serving

1. In a large pot, melt the coconut oil over medium heat. Add the cremini mushrooms, onion and garlic and cook, stirring occasionally, for 5 minutes. Stir in the tarragon, parsley and thyme and continue to cook until the mushrooms are tender, about 5 minutes. Set aside to cool slightly and then transfer to a high-speed blender.

2. Meanwhile, heat the vegetable stock in a medium saucepan over medium-high heat. Carefully pour it into the blender. Add the Italian-Seasoned Ghee and blend until smooth. Transfer the soup to the pot and keep warm over low heat until ready to serve.

3. If using the chanterelle mushrooms, rehydrate them in a small bowl of hot water for a few minutes. Drain the mushrooms and add to the soup.

4. Serve the soup hot, topped with crumbled goat cheese and a drizzle of olive oil. Store, without the goat cheese and olive oil, in an airtight container in the fridge for up to 5 days or in a mason jar in the freezer for up to 3 months.

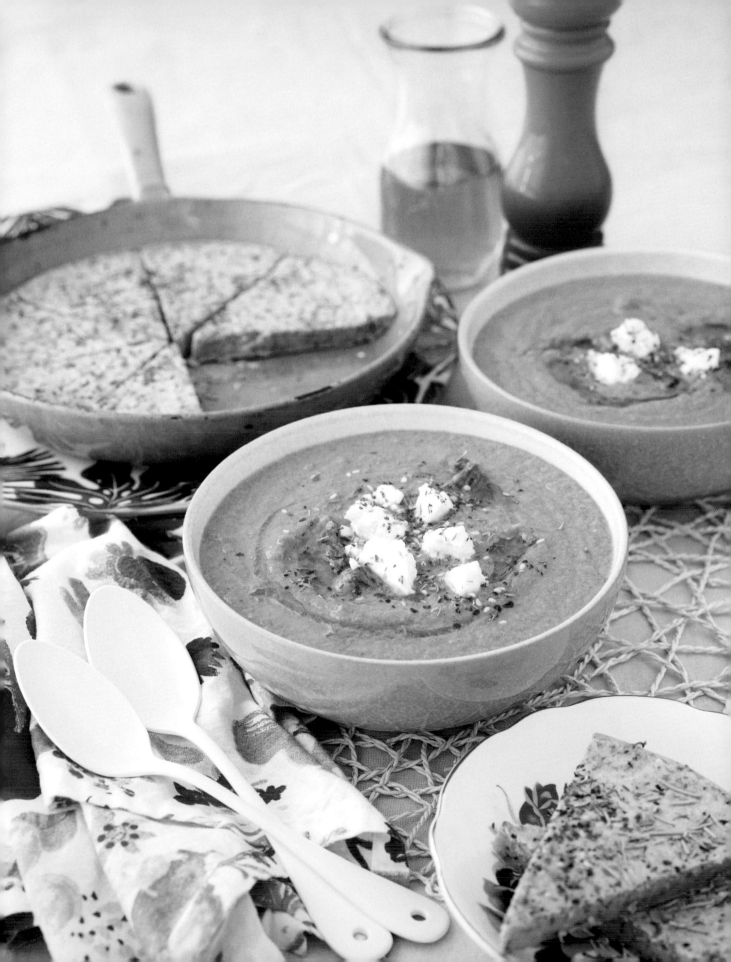

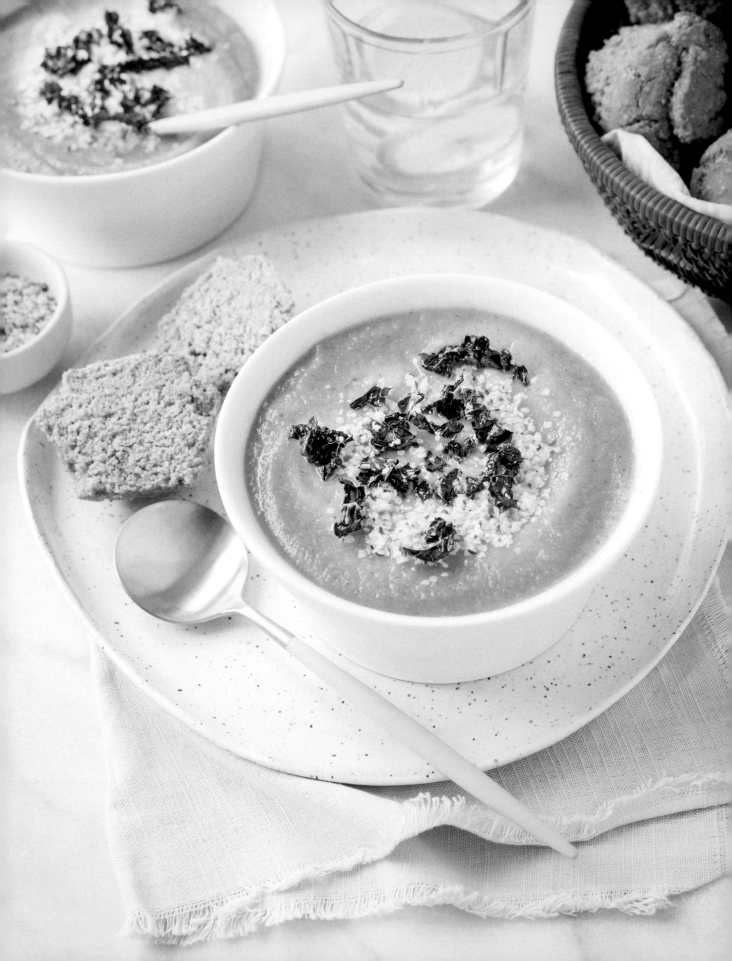

Roasted Pear and Parsnip Soup with Kale Chips

Dairy-free · Gluten-free · Grain-free · Kid-friendly · Nut-free · Vegan

Serves 4 to 6

I didn't grow up eating parsnips, even though they're local to where I lived. They weren't found on my friends' dinner plates either, unless they were mashed and drowned in butter. Parsnips and I found each other when I was an adult, and I fell in love fast because they're a very grounding root veggie. When you add the sweetness of pear to the mix, you've got a match made in heaven. Pear does a lovely job of softening the distinct flavour of parsnip. Top this soup with the crunchy, salty kale chips and you're satisfying all the tastes. This soup is great enjoyed with my Spicy Cornbread Muffins (page 129) made without jalapeño peppers.

Roasted Pear and Parsnip Soup

3 ripe pears (Bosc or Bartlett), cored and roughly chopped
2 cups (500 mL) parsnips cut into chunks
1 small white onion, chopped
3 or 4 cloves garlic, chopped
1 tablespoon (15 mL) extra-virgin olive oil
1 teaspoon (5 mL) dried thyme
3 to 4 cups (750 mL to 1 L) vegetable stock
¼ cup (60 mL) hemp seeds, for garnish

Kale Chips

1 bunch lacinato kale, centre stems removed, chopped into bite-size pieces
1 teaspoon (5 mL) extra-virgin olive oil
Pinch of sea salt

1. **Make the Roasted Pear and Parsnip Soup** Preheat the oven to 350°F (180°C). Line a baking sheet with parchment paper.

2. Place the pears, parsnips, onion and garlic in a large baking dish. Toss together with the olive oil. Sprinkle with the thyme. Cover and roast for 45 to 50 minutes, until the parsnips are fork-tender.

3. Remove the roasted vegetables from the oven and let cool slightly. Leave the oven on to cook the kale chips. Transfer the vegetables to a high-speed blender or food processor and add 3 cups (750 mL) of the vegetable stock. Blend until smooth. Add up to 1 cup (250 mL) stock for a thinner consistency, if needed. Transfer the soup to a large pot and heat over medium heat, then reduce the heat to low and keep warm until ready to serve.

4. **Make the Kale Chips** Spread the kale evenly on the prepared baking sheet. Rub with the olive oil and sprinkle with sea salt. Bake for 8 minutes, or until the kale is crispy. Be careful not to burn it.

5. Serve the soup hot, topped with Kale Chips and a sprinkle of hemp seeds. Store, without the Kale Chips and hemp seeds, in an airtight container in the fridge for up to 5 days or in a mason jar in the freezer for up to 3 months.

Roasted Red Pepper Soup

Dairy-free • Gluten-free • Grain-free • Vegan

Serves 4

Nothing says summer like sweet red pepper soup. Of course I can buy peppers all year round from grocery stores, but shopping at a farmers' market for freshly grown local peppers makes my heart sing! The great thing about sweet peppers is that if you can't find red ones, then orange or yellow will do the trick. This soup is delicious either cold or hot. If it's humid and hot when you make this, refrigerate it for a couple of hours before serving. Add a nice schlop of sour cream or coconut yogurt on top with some fresh herbs from your garden and you have the perfect soup for a summer barbecue with friends. If you're enjoying it on a cold winter's night, then you've got half of the quintessential Canadian meal: serve it with my comforting Grilled Cheese and Pear Sammies (page 187) for a casual dinner with your favourite Netflix series.

6 to 8 sweet red peppers, cut in quarters
2 tablespoons (30 mL) extra-virgin
   olive oil, divided
1 white onion, chopped
2 cloves garlic, finely chopped
1½ to 2 cups (375 to 500 mL)
   vegetable stock, divided
1 teaspoon (5 mL) sea salt

Garnish
Chopped fresh curly parsley
Crumbled dried rosemary
Pine nuts
Plain coconut yogurt (optional)

1. Preheat the oven to 375°F (190°C). Line a baking sheet with parchment paper.

2. Place the red peppers cut side down on the prepared baking sheet and drizzle with 1 tablespoon (15 mL) of the olive oil. Bake for 25 to 30 minutes, until the peppers are fork-tender and slightly blistered. Let cool slightly.

3. Meanwhile, in a large frying pan, heat the remaining 1 tablespoon (15 mL) olive oil over medium heat. Add the onion and garlic and cook, stirring occasionally, until the onions are soft and translucent, about 5 minutes.

4. In a high-speed blender, combine the red peppers, onion mixture, 1½ cups (375 mL) of the vegetable stock and the sea salt. Pulse until smooth. Add up to ½ cup (125 mL) stock for a thinner consistency, if needed. Reheat before serving or refrigerate for a few hours.

5. Serve the soup hot or chilled topped with fresh parsley, dried rosemary, pine nuts and coconut yogurt, if using. Store, without the garnishes, in an airtight container in the fridge for up to 5 days or in a mason jar in the freezer for up to 3 months.

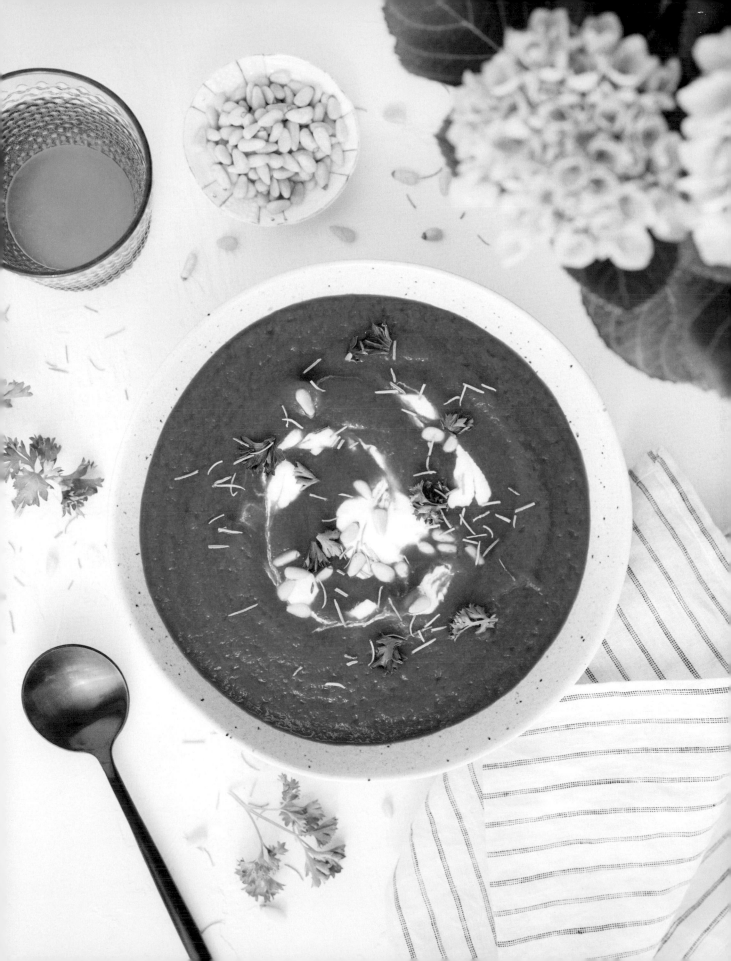

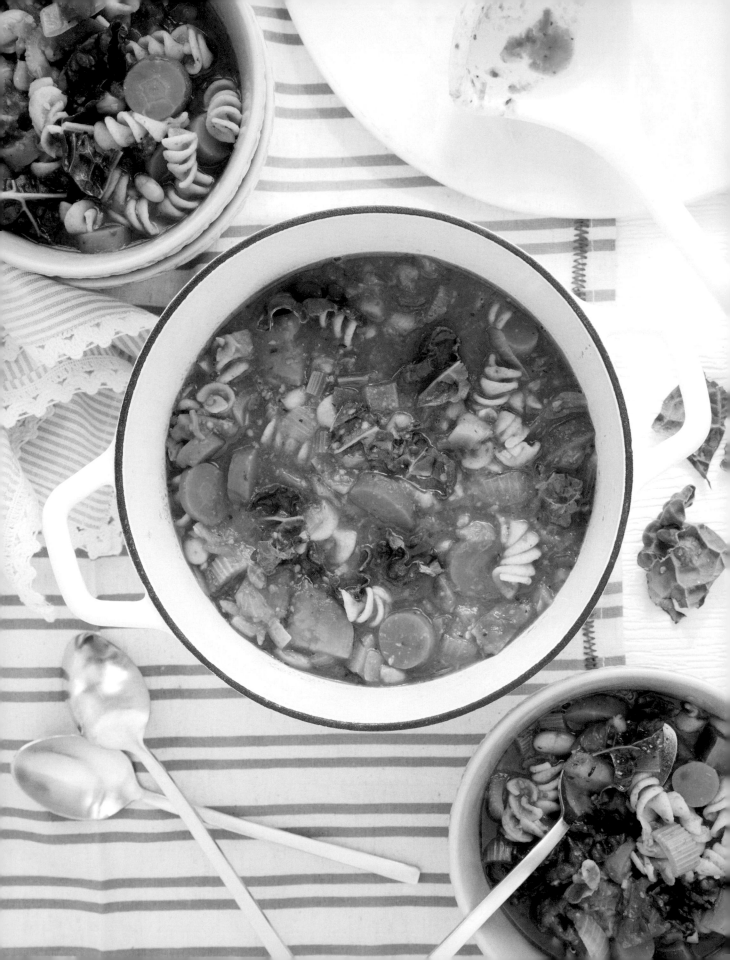

Minestrone Soup
Dairy-free • Kid-friendly • Nut-free • Vegan

Serves 6

When I was a kid, soup was one of those dishes that always made me feel better when I was sick, thanks to my mom. She was and still is the soup queen, and I owe all my soup-making abilities to her. Her vegetable soup, which is essentially a minestrone soup, was the inspiration for this recipe. It's the ultimate healthy comfort food.

   This soup is so packed with nourishing, whole ingredients that it's a meal in itself. This is definitely one of my all-time favourite soups. I hope you love it just as much as I do.

2 tablespoons (30 mL) extra-virgin olive oil

1 white onion, chopped

2 cloves garlic, chopped

4 celery stalks, chopped

4 carrots, sliced into rounds

1 medium zucchini, chopped

2 small sweet potatoes, cubed

1 can (28 ounces/796 mL) whole
   tomatoes, undrained

1 can (14 ounces/398 mL) cannellini
   beans, drained and rinsed

2 tablespoons (30 mL) dried Italian herbs

2 dried bay leaves

1 cup (250 mL) gluten-free or spelt fusilli

3 to 4 cups (750 mL to 1 L) vegetable stock,
   divided

3 kale leaves, centre stems removed and
   roughly chopped

Sea salt and pepper

1. In a large pot, heat the olive oil over medium heat. Add the onion and garlic and cook, stirring occasionally, until the onions are soft and translucent, about 5 minutes.

2. Add the celery, carrots and zucchini and cook, stirring occasionally, for 5 more minutes, until glossy. Add the sweet potatoes, tomatoes and their juice, cannellini beans, Italian herbs and bay leaves. Simmer for 10 minutes.

3. Add the pasta and 3 cups (750 mL) of the vegetable stock. Bring to a gentle boil, then reduce the heat and simmer for 10 minutes. Add up to 1 cup (250 mL) stock for a thinner consistency, if needed.

4. Stir in the chopped kale, then remove the pot from the heat. The kale will wilt quickly. Season with sea salt and pepper. Remove the bay leaves before serving. Store in an airtight container in the fridge for up to 5 days or in a mason jar in the freezer for up to 3 months.

Butternut Squash Lentil Soup

Dairy-free • Gluten-free • Grain-free • Kid-friendly • Nut-free

Serves 6

This wonderfully nourishing soup is cozy and warming to the whole body. It's easily an entire meal because the lentils are hearty and rich in protein and fibre. I prefer sprouted lentils because they are easier on the digestive system and their nutrients are more easily absorbed. But of course you can use regular lentils. And adding butternut squash just makes everything taste good.

I often make this soup on the weekend so I know I'll have a healthy weekday lunch for the busy week ahead. Enjoy it with my Mushroom, Asparagus and Feta Tartines (page 122).

1 tablespoon (15 mL) coconut oil
1 large white onion, chopped
2 cloves garlic, finely chopped
1 butternut squash, peeled, seeded and cubed
2 cups (500 mL) green lentils, preferably sprouted
4 to 6 cups (1 to 1.5 L) chicken or vegetable stock, divided
1 teaspoon (5 mL) dried tarragon
1 can (14 ounces/400 mL) full-fat coconut milk
4 kale leaves, centre stems removed, chopped

1. In a large pot, melt the coconut oil over medium heat. Add the onion and garlic and cook, stirring occasionally, until the onions are soft and translucent, about 5 minutes. (If using a slow cooker, cook the onions in a large frying pan, then transfer them to the slow cooker.)

2. Add the butternut squash, lentils, 4 cups (1 L) of the chicken stock and the tarragon. Bring to a boil over high heat, then reduce the heat and simmer for 15 to 20 minutes, until the squash is fork-tender. Add up to 2 cups (500 mL) stock if the soup is getting too thick or if you want a thinner consistency. (If using a slow cooker, set for 2 hours.)

3. Once the lentils are cooked and the squash is fork-tender, stir in the coconut milk and chopped kale. Serve immediately or store in an airtight container in the fridge for up to 5 days or in a mason jar in the freezer for up to 3 months.

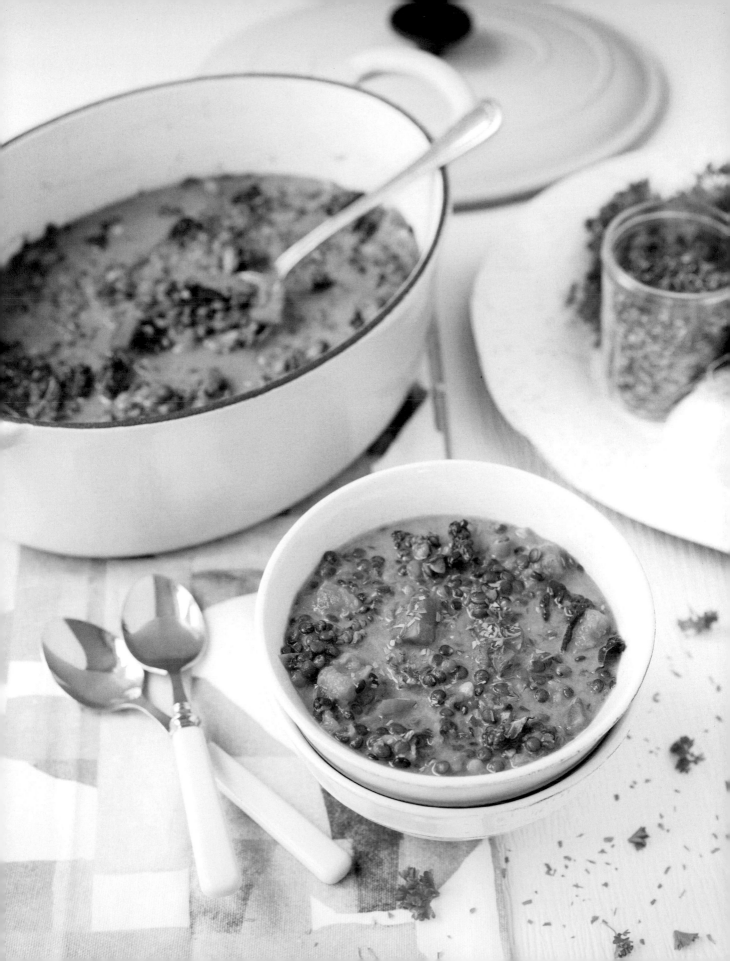

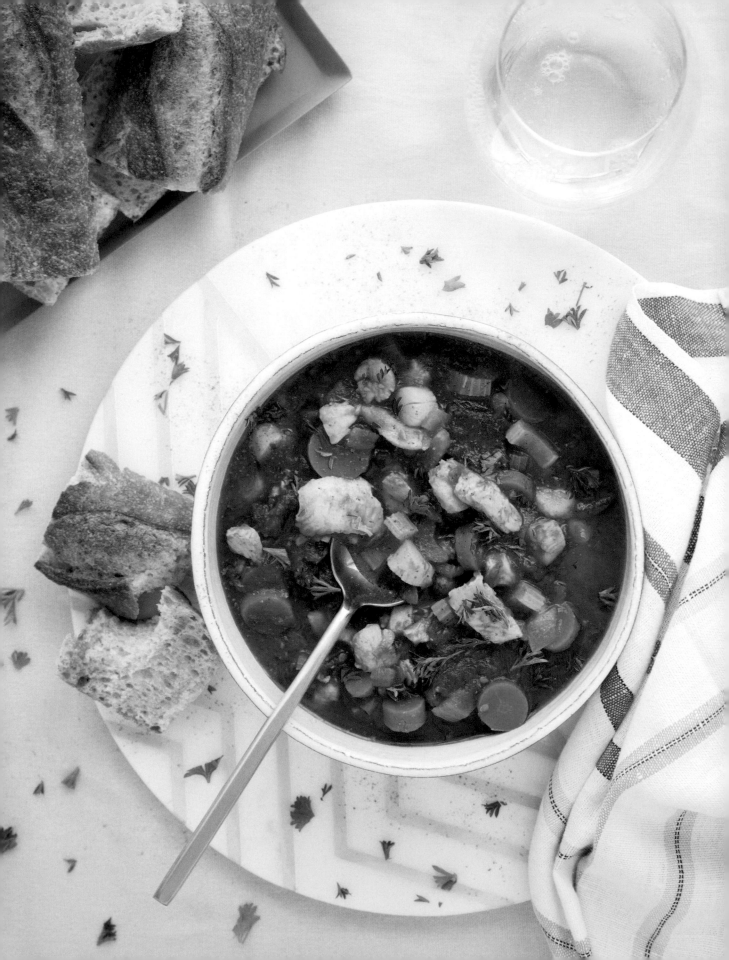

Mamabea's Seafood Soup

Dairy-free • Gluten-free • Grain-free • Nut-free

Serves 4

I remember the first time I had this soup like it was yesterday. We were at Walker's grandma's house—everyone calls her Mamabea. It was a cold, snowy afternoon and I was pregnant, so basically I was hungry 24/7. This soup warmed me from the inside out and nourished me well. I remember I kept saying, "This is so delicious!" If you love seafood, you are going to love this soup.

You can easily double the recipe if you are serving a crowd. If you want to turn it into a stew, reduce the liquid by cooking it a bit longer before adding the seafood. Or add a bit of water for a thinner consistency. If you're making this with limited time on your hands, you can toss both the sole and the scallops in frozen. I let the sole thaw a little bit and then use scissors to cut it into chunks, but it's still pretty frozen when I add it. Just let them simmer a little longer to make sure they're cooked through.

2 tablespoons (30 mL) extra-virgin olive oil or coconut oil
1 medium white onion, chopped
1 to 2 cloves garlic, chopped
3 carrots, chopped
3 celery stalks, chopped
1 can (28 ounces/796 mL) whole tomatoes, undrained
½ cup (125 mL) dry white wine
3 fresh or thawed frozen sole fillets, cut into cubes
1 cup (250 mL) fresh or thawed frozen scallops
Zest of 1 orange
1 tablespoon (15 mL) dried tarragon
½ teaspoon (2 mL) sea salt
Pinch of saffron (optional)
¼ cup (60 mL) loosely packed chopped fresh curly parsley, for garnish

1. In a large pot, heat the olive oil over medium heat. Add the onion and garlic and cook, stirring occasionally, until the onions are soft and translucent, about 5 minutes.

2. Add the carrots and celery and cook for 5 more minutes. Add the tomatoes and their juice and white wine and cook for 10 minutes.

3. Add the sole, scallops, orange zest, tarragon, sea salt and saffron, if using. Simmer for 10 more minutes, or until the sole and scallops are just cooked through. Serve hot, garnished with the parsley. Store in airtight container in the fridge for up to 3 days.

Homemade Tomato Sauce

Dairy-free • Gluten-free • Grain-free • Kid-friendly • Nut-free • Vegan

Makes 6 cups (1.5 L)

When local tomatoes are abundant at farmers' markets, my hubs, Walker, and I rejoice because we can make our own sauce. You just can't beat the flavour and texture of homemade tomato sauce! This recipe is a blank canvas—let your creativity run free when it comes to adding spices and vegetables. I prefer everything as fresh as possible, so I freeze the basic sauce in batches and add other ingredients when I heat it up. For instance, I'll add fresh garlic and fresh basil if I'm serving the sauce with zucchini noodles or pasta.

You might be wondering why I don't remove the seeds or the skins in this recipe. That's because there are no rules with this recipe! There's no reason to remove them, and it speeds things up too. If you prefer a thicker sauce, you can easily reduce it down on the stovetop or you can add some tomato paste. I love using this sauce in my Zucchini Noodles with Turkey Meatballs (page 196) and my Super-Quick Tortilla Pizzas (page 175)!

24 Roma or field tomatoes, washed

1. Preheat the oven to 350°F (180°C). Line a baking sheet with parchment paper.

2. Slice the tomatoes in half lengthwise and arrange them cut side down on the prepared baking sheet. Bake for 30 to 40 minutes, until the tomatoes are slightly blistered but not burnt. Let cool slightly.

3. Transfer the tomato halves to a high-speed blender and blend until smooth. Store in airtight containers in the fridge for up to 5 days or in mason jars in the freezer for up to 3 months.

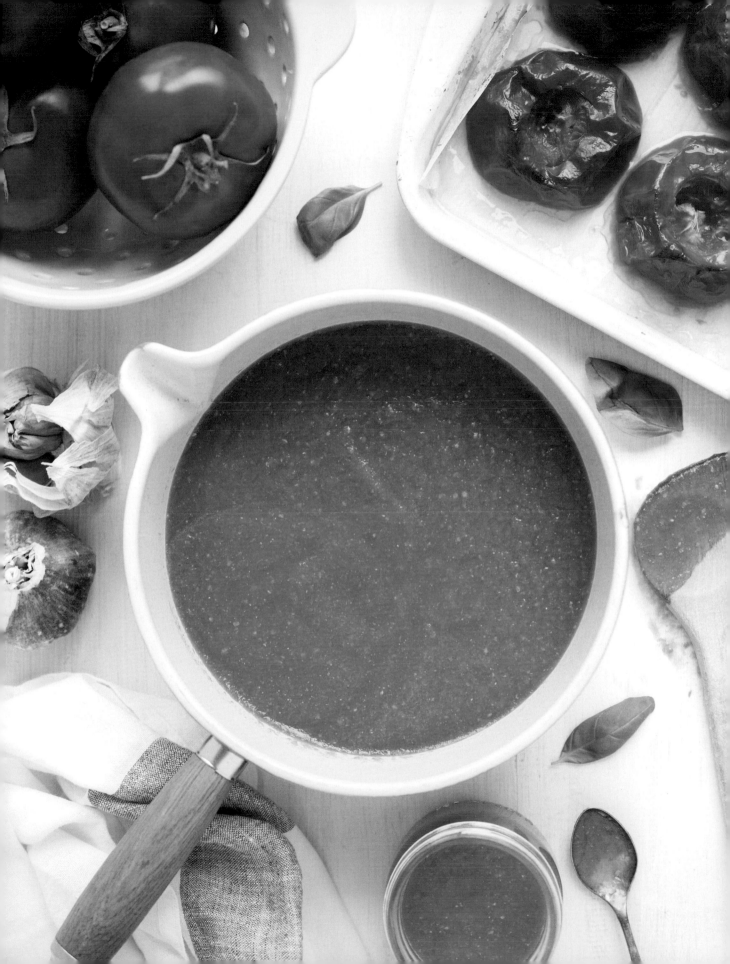

Veggies and Shrimp Green Curry

Dairy-free • Gluten-free • Nut-free

Serves 4

Throughout my childhood my dad enjoyed slow cooking on the weekends, making dishes like chilies and his mouthwatering chowders. Cooking was definitely a happy place for him, and I know this because when my dad cooked he whistled, and he always whistled when he was focused and enjoying something.

Although my dad never followed a recipe, I eventually managed to get him to write down the recipe for his seafood chowder for me, and since then it has morphed into this green curry—a favourite in my home because it is full of rich flavours and incredibly filling. Serve my Veggie Rolls with Spicy Almond Sauce (page 125) as a starter.

The arrowroot starch helps to make the broth nice and thick, but you can skip it if your broth is creamy enough from the coconut milk.

1 cup (250 mL) short-grain brown rice
2 cups (500 mL) water
1 tablespoon (15 mL) coconut oil
½ large white onion, finely chopped
1 to 2 cloves garlic, finely chopped
1 cup (250 mL) cremini or white button mushrooms, chopped in large chunks
2 cups (500 mL) cauliflower florets
½ large sweet yellow pepper, sliced lengthwise
1 cup (250 mL) sugar snap peas
2 cans (14 ounces/400 mL each) full-fat coconut milk
8 to 12 fresh or thawed frozen medium shrimp (about 8 ounces/225 g), peeled
3 tablespoons (45 mL) Thai green curry paste
2 tablespoons (30 mL) arrowroot starch/flour (optional)
¼ cup (60 mL) tightly packed chopped fresh cilantro

1. In a medium saucepan, combine the rice and water and bring to a boil over high heat. Reduce the heat to low, cover and cook for 25 to 30 minutes, until the rice is tender. Remove from the heat and fluff with a fork. Keep warm.

2. Meanwhile, melt the coconut oil in a large pot over medium heat. Add the onion and garlic and cook, stirring occasionally, until the onions are soft and translucent, about 5 minutes. Add the mushrooms and cook for another 5 minutes. Add the cauliflower, yellow pepper and sugar snap peas and cook for 5 more minutes.

3. Stir in the coconut milk. Add the shrimp and cook for 3 to 4 minutes, just until pink and plump. Stir in the green curry paste.

4. If you'd like your soup a bit thicker, in a small bowl, whisk together the arrowroot starch and ¼ cup (60 mL) water and add to the pot. You can skip this step if the soup is already creamy enough.

5. Remove from the heat and let the flavours mingle for 5 minutes with the lid on. Serve hot over the brown rice and garnish with cilantro. Store in an airtight container in the fridge for up to 3 days.

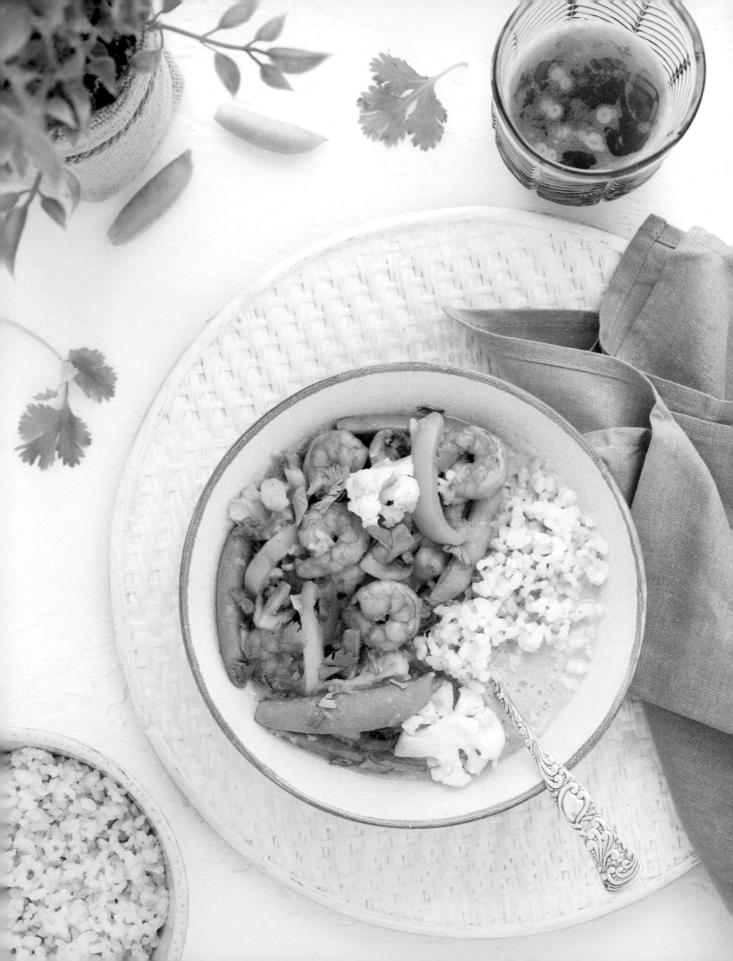

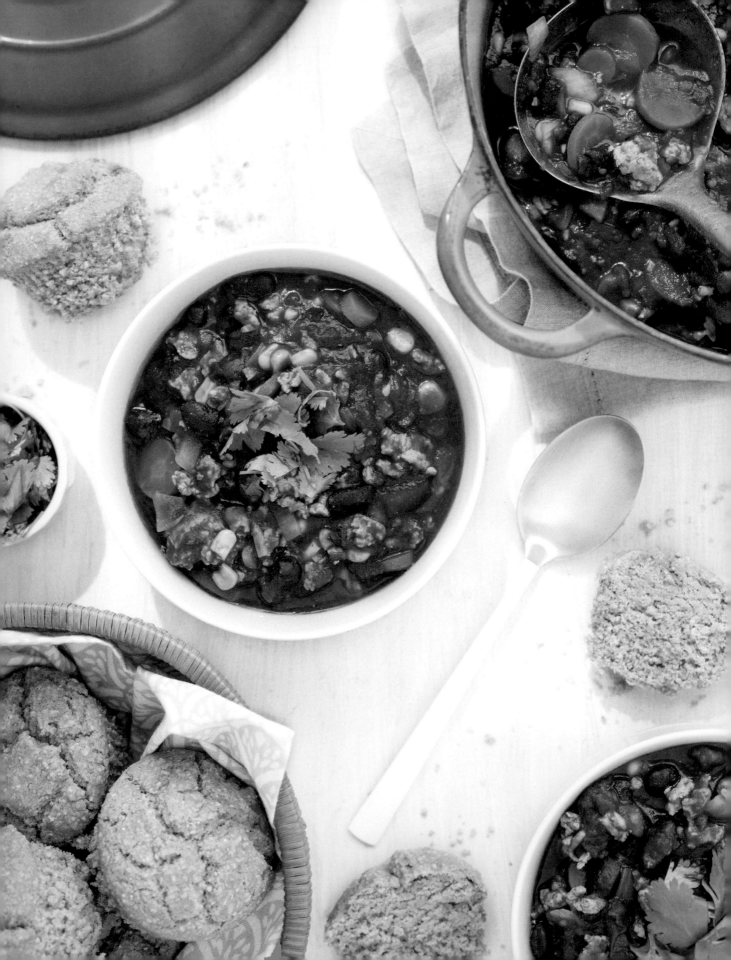

Slow Cooker Spicy Turkey Chili

Dairy-free • Gluten-free • Grain-free • Kid-friendly • Nut-free

Serves 8

My good friend Patrick makes a mean chili, so when he kindly offered to share his recipe, I jumped at the chance to include it in the cookbook. My family loves it, and it reminds me of the chili my dad used to make on weekends when I was growing up. The only thing I added—but I'm sure Pat would approve—is the carrots, just to beef up the vegetables.

This is a great recipe for when you have a big crowd to feed or if you want to make a large batch to enjoy leftovers. Chili freezes really well, making it ideal for easy weeknight dinners. If you don't have a slow cooker you can simply make the chili in a large soup pot; the slow cooking is really just to allow the flavours to mingle. And if you let it sit overnight, it tastes even better the next day. If you're making this for young ones, you might want to leave out the jalapeño and cayenne pepper so it's not too spicy! Enjoy with my Spicy Cornbread Muffins (page 129), with or without the jalapeño.

2 tablespoons (30 mL) extra-virgin olive oil
2 pounds (900 g) ground organic turkey
   or chicken
1 large white onion, finely chopped
4 carrots, sliced into rounds
5 to 6 cloves garlic, chopped
2 jalapeño peppers, seeded and finely
   chopped
1 sweet red pepper, chopped
1 cup (250 mL) frozen corn kernels
1 tablespoon (15 mL) ground cumin
1 to 2 teaspoons (5 to 10 mL) cayenne
   pepper
2 cans (14 ounces/398 mL each) kidney
   beans, drained and rinsed
2 cans (28 ounces/796 mL each) whole
   tomatoes, undrained
1 can (5½ ounces/156 mL) tomato paste

1. In a large frying pan, heat the olive oil over medium heat. Add the ground turkey and cook, stirring frequently, until no longer pink, 10 to 12 minutes. Add to the slow cooker. (Alternatively, cook the turkey in a large pot.)

2. Add the onion, carrots, garlic, jalapeños, red pepper, corn, cumin, cayenne, kidney beans, tomatoes and their juice, and tomato paste. Stir to combine. Cook on low for 6 to 7 hours. (If cooking in a pot, simmer for 1 to 2 hours.)

3. Store in an airtight container in the fridge for up to 5 days or in a mason jars in the freezer for up to 3 months.

One-Pot Paprika Chicken
Dairy-free • Gluten-free • Grain-free • Nut-free

Serves 4

Every summer we visit my father-in-law in Austria, and when we eat out at restaurants pretty much every warm dish contains paprika. Yes, we eat a lot of goulash, and paprika is its signature ingredient. I love how easy this dish is to pull together on a chilly winter night. It's so flavourful, hearty and filling—the perfect meal to warm your soul without too much fuss or mess, just the way a one-pot meal should be.

You can enjoy this over some pasta or, as we do, with my Creamy Kale and Apricot Salad with Roasted Chickpeas (page 107) on the side.

2 tablespoons (30 mL) extra-virgin olive oil

2 white onions, finely chopped

2 cloves garlic, finely chopped

1 to 2 teaspoons (5 to 10 mL) sweet paprika

1 teaspoon (5 mL) ground cumin

4 boneless, skinless organic chicken breasts, cut in half crosswise

2 cans (28 ounces/796 mL each) diced tomatoes, undrained

½ cup (125 mL) Kalamata olives, preferably with pits for flavour

¼ cup (60 mL) chopped fresh basil or curly parsley, for garnish

1. In a large saucepan, heat the olive oil over medium heat. Add the onions, garlic, paprika and cumin and cook, stirring occasionally, until the onions are soft and translucent, about 5 minutes.

2. Add the chicken, tomatoes and their juice, and olives. Boil gently for 3 minutes. Reduce the heat and simmer for 20 to 25 minutes, until the chicken is fully cooked and the sauce has thickened.

3. Serve hot, garnished with basil. Store in an airtight container in the fridge for up to 5 days or in a mason jar in the freezer for up to 3 months.

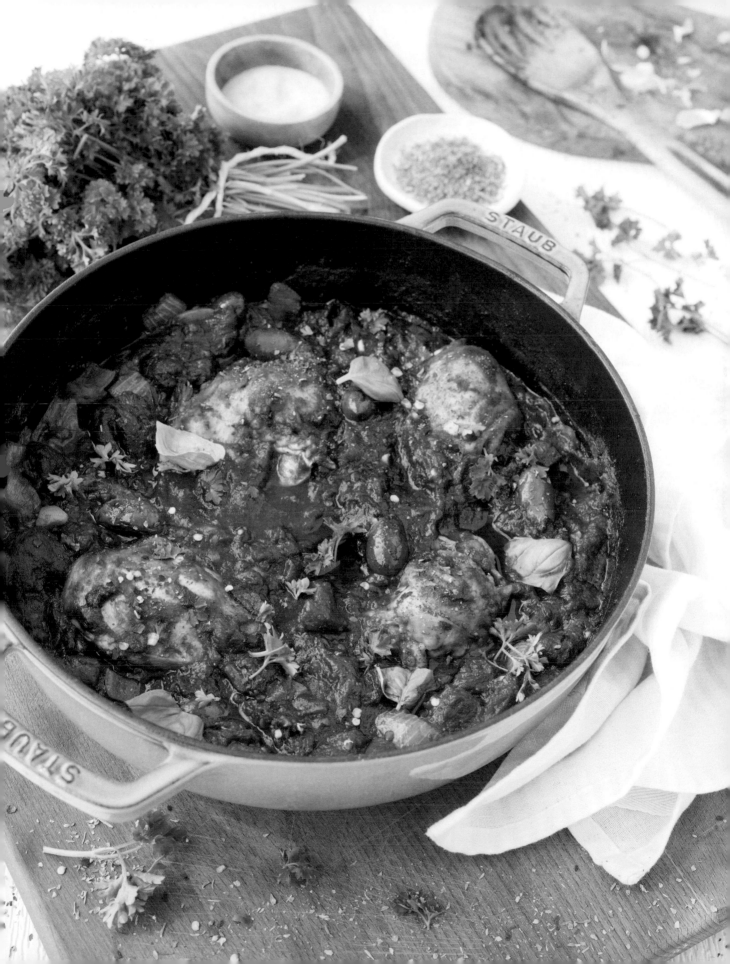

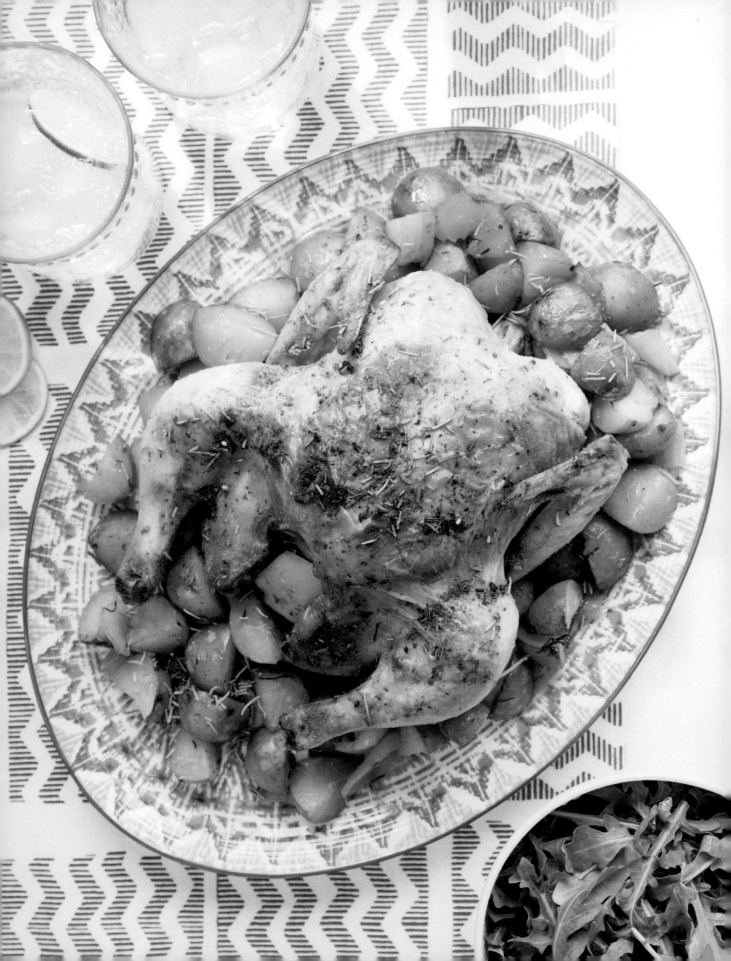

Rosemary and Thyme Roasted Chicken with Baby Potatoes

Gluten-free • Grain-free • Kid-friendly • Nut-free

Serves 4

I love roasting a whole chicken partly because my entire kitchen smells so delicious! Of course there are more reasons to roast a whole chicken than just the smell. It's very comforting to do early on a Sunday evening when I have no plans other than hanging out with my family waiting for a delicious meal to unfold with next to no effort. Once a bit of prep is done, the oven does all the work.

This roasted chicken with rosemary and baby potatoes needs nothing more than a side dish of Garlicky Green Beans with Tahini Lemon Sauce (page 118) and a few hungry people to gobble up every morsel. I love sliced leftover roast chicken in salads and wraps the next day. In fact, leftovers are a lovely addition to my Grilled Cheese and Pear Sammies (page 187).

1 whole organic chicken
   (about 3½ pounds/1.6 kg)
1 medium white onion, roughly chopped
1 lemon, cut into chunks
4 cups (1 L) baby white potatoes,
   cut in half
5 tablespoons (75 mL) Original Ghee
   (page 43) or store-bought ghee
4 cloves garlic, chopped
1 tablespoon (15 mL) dried rosemary
1 tablespoon (15 mL) dried thyme
Sea salt and pepper

1. Preheat the oven to 400°F (200°C).

2. Place the chicken in a large roasting pan and stuff with the chopped onions and lemon. Tie the legs together with twine if you like (I don't bother). Spread the potatoes evenly around the chicken.

3. Melt the Original Ghee in a small pot over medium heat. Stir in the garlic, rosemary and thyme. Pour the mixture over the chicken and season with sea salt and pepper.

4. Roast for 45 minutes. Remove from the oven and spoon the juices over the chicken and potatoes. Return to the oven and roast for another 30 minutes, or until the chicken juices run clear. You can also use a meat thermometer inserted in the thick part of the thigh without touching the bone. The chicken is done when the temperature is 165°F (74°C). Transfer the chicken to a cutting board and let rest for 10 minutes.

5. Meanwhile, if you'd like to crisp up the potatoes a bit, return the pan to the oven and roast for another 5 to 10 minutes.

6. Using a carving knife, slice the chicken and place on a serving platter with the potatoes.

Baked Chicken with Dijon Maple Marinade

Dairy-free • Gluten-free • Grain-free • Kid-friendly • Nut-free

Serves 4

I used to think chicken thighs were unhealthy, but I was mistaken. The good fat is amazing for healthy skin and hair! Not only are they healthy, but chicken thighs are the tastiest part of the chicken, in my opinion. They are always juicy and they are very versatile. I sometimes use them in my One-Pot Paprika Chicken (page 162) when I want to change up the recipe from chicken breasts or if there's a sale on organic chicken thighs at the grocery store.

Dijon mustard, maple syrup and chicken were meant to be together. If you like a more saucy dish so that you can scoop up the sauce with a spoon, simply double the marinade. This dish pairs nicely with the richness of my Roasted Root Veggies (page 116).

2 pounds (900 g) organic bone-in,
   skin-on chicken thighs
2 cloves garlic, finely chopped
¼ cup (60 mL) Dijon mustard
3 tablespoons (45 mL) real maple syrup
2 tablespoons (30 mL) extra-virgin olive oil
2 tablespoons (30 mL) filtered water
1 teaspoon (5 mL) dried tarragon
Sea salt and pepper

1. Place the chicken thighs skin side up in a large baking dish. In a small bowl, whisk together the garlic, mustard, maple syrup, olive oil, water and tarragon. Pour the marinade over the chicken and let sit in the fridge for 1 to 2 hours.

2. Preheat the oven to 350°F (180°C).

3. Bake the chicken for 35 to 40 minutes, until the juices run clear. Season with sea salt and pepper. Enjoy immediately.

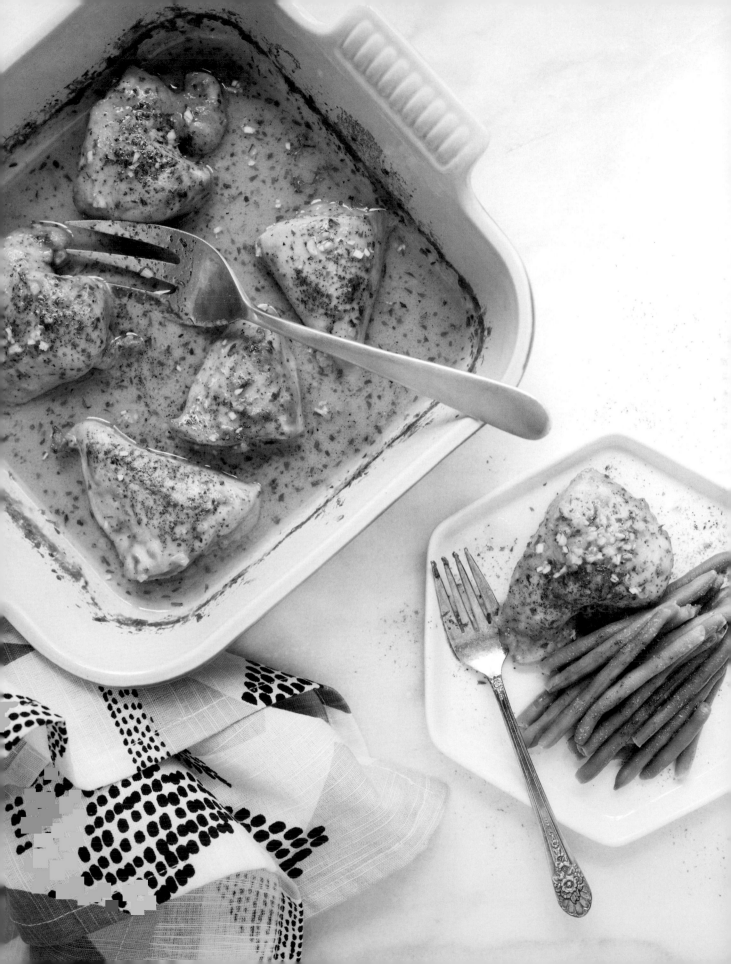

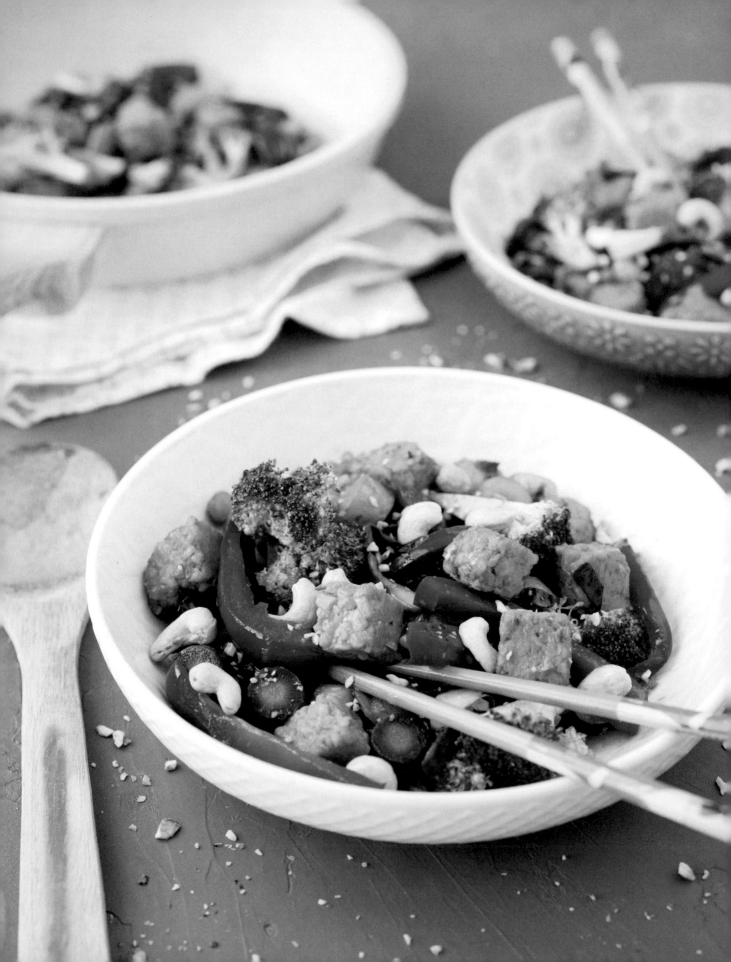

Tempeh Veggie Stir-Fry with Ginger Tamari Sauce

Dairy-free • Gluten-free • Grain-free • Vegan

Serves 4

Tempeh is an ideal source of plant-based protein because it has all the essential amino acids, which is why it's such a popular choice with vegans and vegetarians. It is so earthy and meaty, and I love it! It's like a chameleon because it takes on the flavours of whatever you cook it with. I make this recipe throughout the year because in the summer I love using local veggies and in the winter it's a meal with substance—stick-to-your-ribs, as they say! Leftovers are great for lunch the next day.

When purchasing tempeh, buy plain and look for "organic" on the label. The majority of soy grown in the world is genetically modified, and GMO crops are often sprayed with more pesticides. Choosing organic means you avoid GMO foods.

Ginger Tamari Sauce

3 cloves garlic, chopped
2 tablespoons (30 mL) grated fresh ginger
½ cup (125 mL) extra-virgin olive oil
¼ cup (60 mL) gluten-free tamari
2 tablespoons (30 mL) real maple syrup
Juice of 1 lime
1 tablespoon (15 mL) arrowroot starch/flour

Tempeh Veggie Stir-Fry

1 package (8 ounces/225 g) organic tempeh, cubed
2 tablespoons (30 mL) coconut oil
1 small white onion, chopped
1 cup (250 mL) chopped carrots
1 sweet red pepper, sliced lengthwise
2 cups (500 mL) broccoli florets
1 cup (250 mL) finely chopped purple cabbage
⅓ cup (75 mL) whole raw cashews
¼ cup (60 mL) crushed raw pistachios

1. **Make the Ginger Tamari Sauce** In a small bowl, combine the garlic, ginger, olive oil, tamari, maple syrup and lime juice.

2. **Make the Tempeh Veggie Stir-Fry** Place the tempeh cubes in a medium bowl. Pour half of the Ginger Tamari Sauce over the tempeh and let marinate at room temperature for 2 to 4 hours. Set aside the remaining Ginger Tamari Sauce for the stir-fry.

3. In a large frying pan, heat the coconut oil over medium heat. Add the onion and cook, stirring occasionally, for 5 minutes. Add the carrots and cook for 5 more minutes. Add the pepper, broccoli and cabbage and cook for 5 more minutes.

4. Stir the arrowroot starch into the reserved Ginger Tamari Sauce and add to the vegetable mixture, then stir in the tempeh and the marinade. Continue to cook, stirring, until heated through and the sauce has coated everything and started to thicken a little. Serve immediately, topped with the cashews and pistachios.

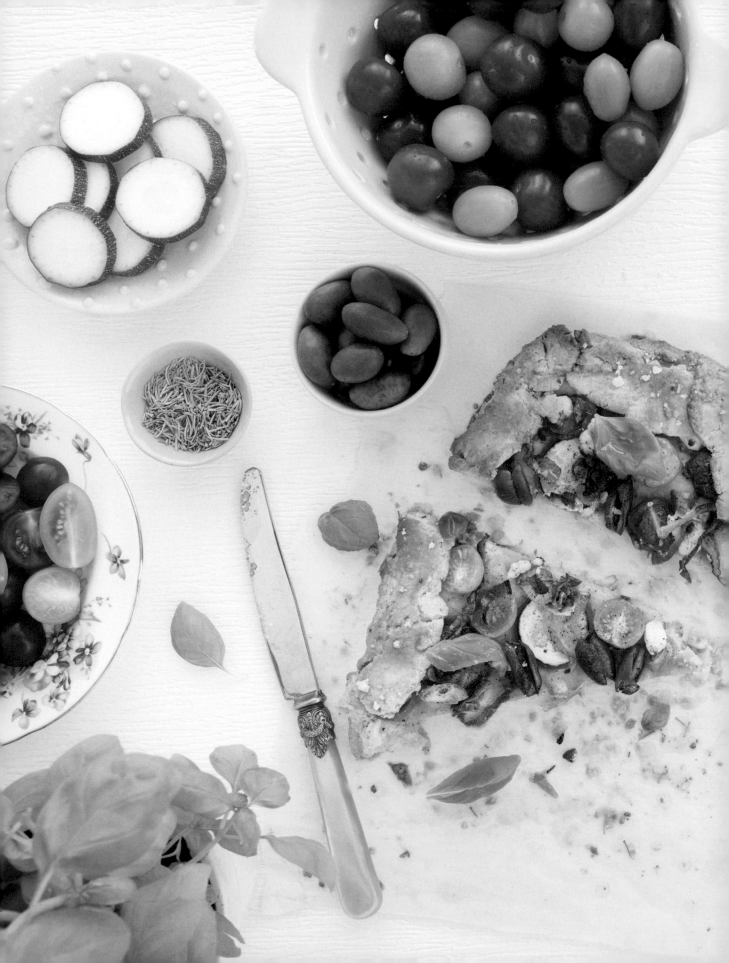

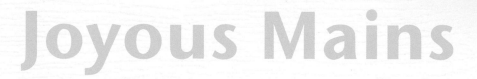

Joyous Mains

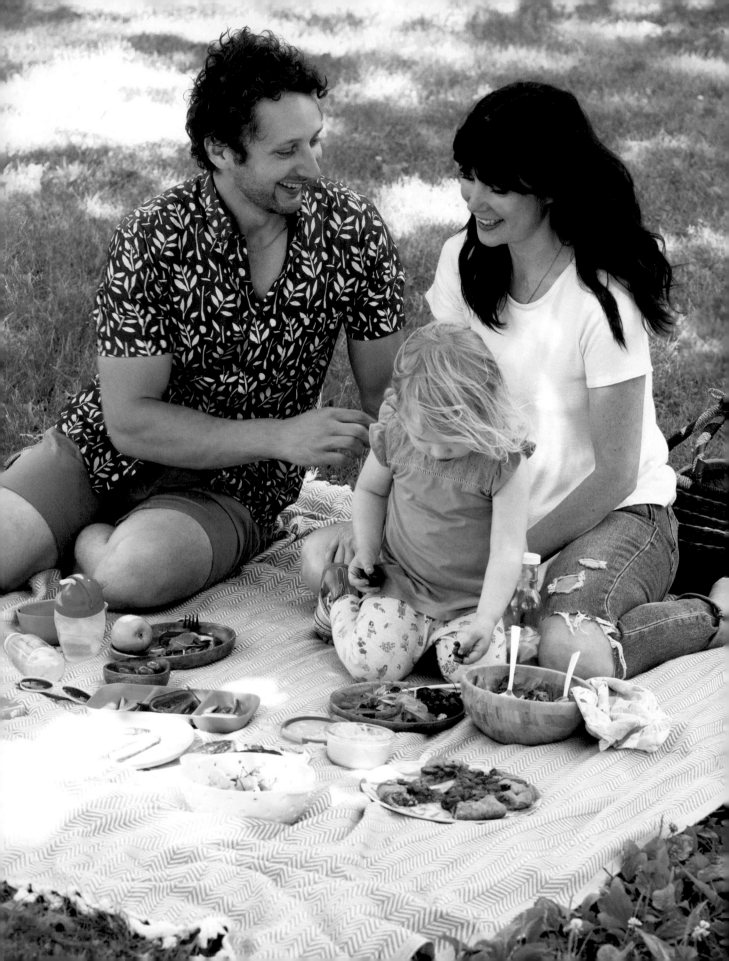

JOYOUS MAINS

It's no secret I love cooking. Whether I'm testing out a new recipe for my blog, experimenting with something I picked up at the farmers' market or spending a typical evening cooking for my loved ones, cooking is my happy place. Making dinner with my little sous-chef Vienna makes it even more enjoyable, even if the kitchen looks like a tornado came through once we are done! I plan out the week's main meals on the weekend and then do most of my grocery shopping at my local health food store. Then we make at least one farmers' market visit to stock up on local fresh produce. There are quite a few markets in our area that run year-round, so we're lucky we can shop all through the seasons.

This chapter contains many of the recipes we return to again and again for lunches and dinners. Now that we have a little one, I make sure my recipes are kid-friendly too. It's easy to get stuck in a rut with main meals, especially when you're super busy during the week, so I hope you find recipes in this chapter that help you change things up and that you find some favourites to come back to. Some of our weeknight go-to dishes are Super-Quick Tortilla Pizzas (page 175) and Crispy Chicken Fingers with Barbecue Sauce (page 176). When we are entertaining, the Rustic Mediterranean Summer Galette (page 199) and the Zucchini Noodles with Turkey Meatballs (page 196) are always a huge hit!

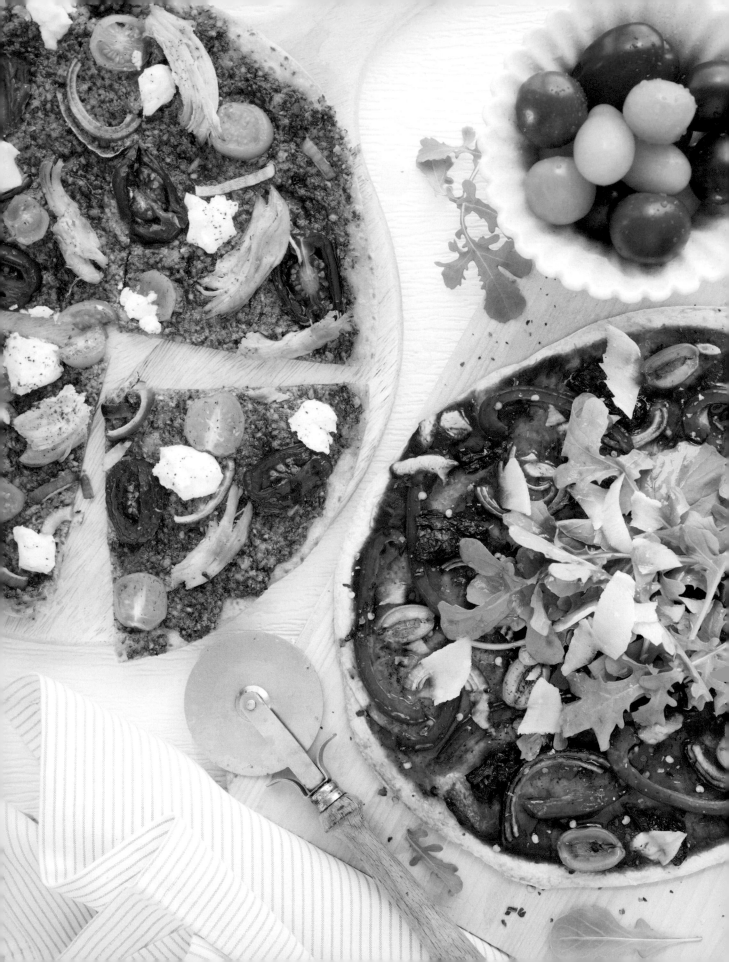

Super-Quick Tortilla Pizzas

Each variation serves 2

Pizza is a favourite in our home. We eat it a few times a month, maybe more! It's a quick, satisfying weeknight meal, and we make it a variety of ways, depending on who's over for dinner or what's in the fridge. The Chicken Pesto Pizza is an entire meal and very filling because of the protein from the chicken, and it's my favourite. It's a perfect way to use up leftovers from Rosemary and Thyme Roasted Chicken (page 165). If you're serving the Veggie Marinara Pizza, then enjoy it with a salad. The Shredded Brussels Sprouts Bean Salad (page 100) is a perfect side to these yummy pizzas.

Chicken Pesto Pizza
Kid-friendly

1 large gluten-free or whole wheat tortilla
½ cup (125 mL) Spinach Walnut Pesto
   (page 192)
2½ ounces (70 g) soft unripened goat
   cheese
½ cup (125 mL) roasted organic chicken
   torn into bite-size pieces
½ cup (125 mL) halved cherry tomatoes
¼ small red onion, thinly sliced

1. Preheat the oven to 350°F (180°C). Line a baking sheet with parchment paper.

2. Place the tortilla on the baking sheet. Evenly spread the Spinach Walnut Pesto over the tortilla, stopping about 1 inch (2.5 cm) from the edge. Sprinkle the goat cheese evenly over the pesto, then top with the chicken, cherry tomatoes and red onions. Bake for 10 to 12 minutes, until the edges are golden and the crust is crisp.

Veggie Marinara Pizza
Kid-friendly • Nut-free • Vegetarian

1 large gluten-free or whole wheat tortilla
½ cup (125 mL) Homemade Tomato Sauce
   (page 156)
5 pitted green olives, cut in half
5 oil-packed sun-dried tomatoes, sliced
¼ small red onion, thinly sliced
½ sweet red pepper, thinly sliced
1 cup (250 mL) loosely packed fresh
   arugula
Shaved Parmesan cheese or 1 tablespoon
   (15 mL) nutritional yeast

1. Preheat the oven to 350°F (180°C). Line a baking sheet with parchment paper.

2. Place the tortilla on the baking sheet. Evenly spread the Homemade Tomato Sauce over the tortilla, stopping about 1 inch (2.5cm) from the edge. Sprinkle the olives, sun-dried tomatoes, red onion and red pepper evenly over the sauce. Bake for 10 to 12 minutes, until the edges are golden and the crust is crisp. Top with arugula and Parmesan.

Crispy Chicken Fingers with Barbecue Sauce

Dairy-free • Gluten-free • Grain-free • Kid-friendly

Serves 4 to 6

What kid and kid-at-heart doesn't love chicken fingers! But too often they're the deep-fried variety, which aren't the healthiest. My chicken fingers are just as crispy and flavourful as their deep-fried counterparts, but they are made with nourishing, whole ingredients. My daughter, Vienna, loves them, and I can feel good about feeding them to her. This recipe has become a staple in our home.

If you have a nut allergy in your home, replace the ground nuts with dried bread crumbs. Serve these with my Curry Sweet Potato Wedges with Yogurt Dill Dip (page 121).

1 cup (250 mL) raw pumpkin seeds
1 cup (250 mL) almond flour
   (almond meal) or ground raw cashews
2 teaspoons (10 mL) garlic powder
2 teaspoons (10 mL) onion powder
½ teaspoon (2 mL) sea salt
2 eggs
4 boneless, skinless organic chicken breasts,
   cut into strips
Paprika Barbecue Sauce (page 204)

1. Preheat the oven to 425°F (220°C). Grease a baking sheet or line with parchment paper.

2. In a food processor, process the pumpkin seeds until crumbly. Transfer to a medium bowl and add the almond flour, garlic powder, onion powder and sea salt. Stir well.

3. In a small bowl, whisk the eggs.

4. Working with one chicken strip at a time, with one hand dip the chicken into the whisked egg, letting the excess drip off. Add it to the seed mixture, and using your other hand, dredge the chicken strip in the mixture to coat. Place the chicken strip on the prepared baking sheet. Repeat with the remaining chicken strips.

5. Bake for 10 minutes, until crispy and golden on the bottom. Turn the chicken strips and bake for another 10 minutes, until crispy and golden on the other side. Serve immediately with Paprika Barbecue Sauce.

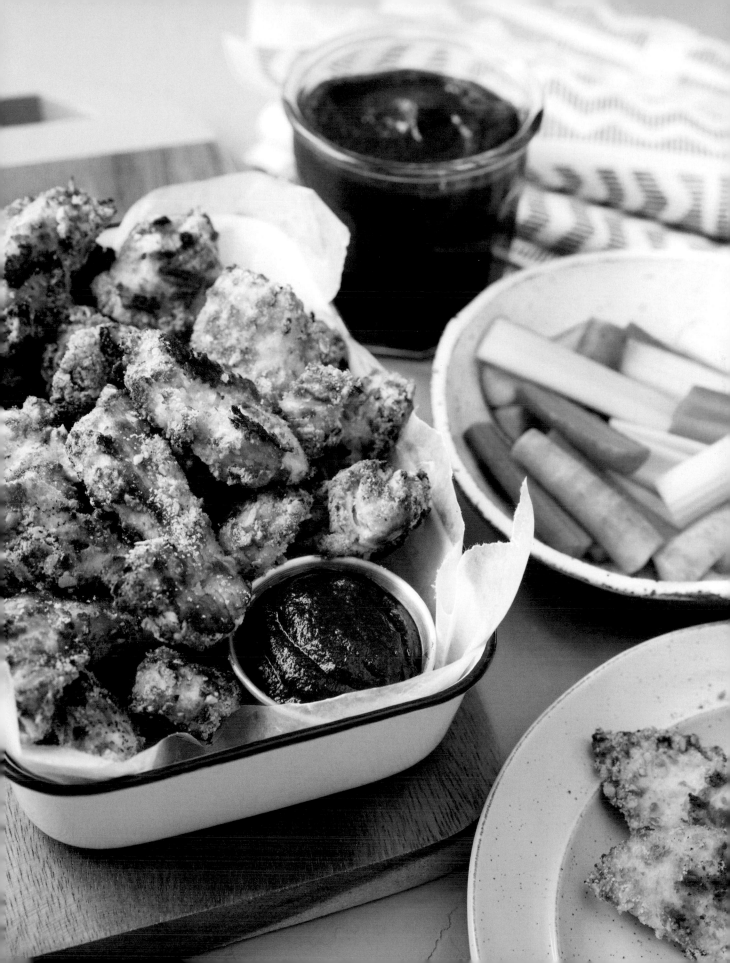

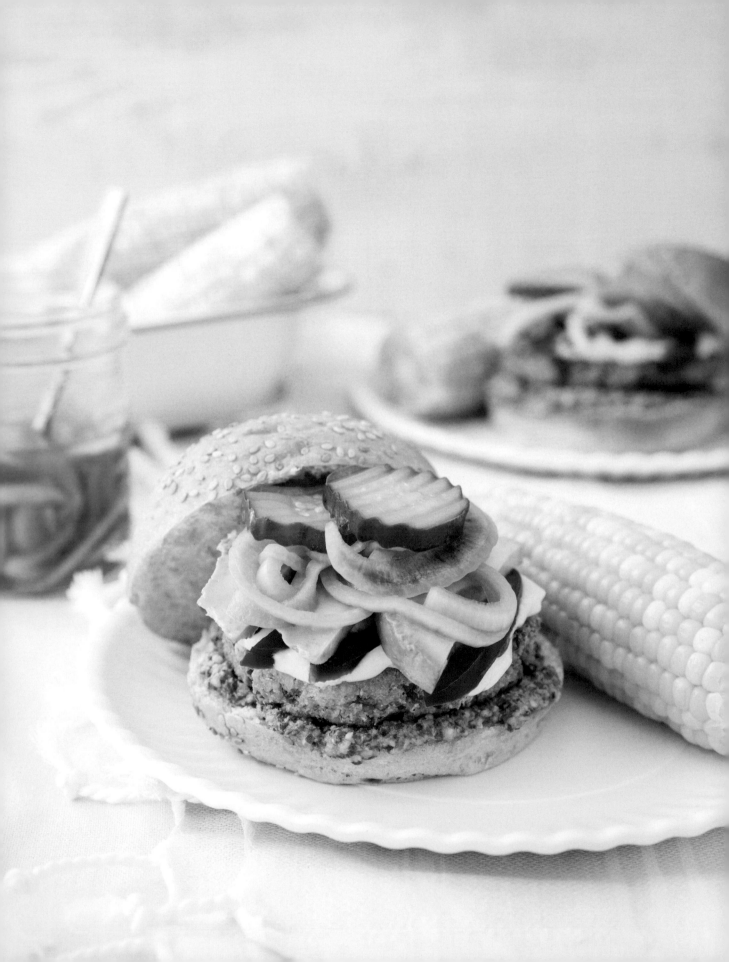

Herby Tempeh Burgers

Dairy-free • Gluten-free • Kid-friendly • Vegetarian

Makes 4 burgers

I love these burgers and we make them year-round, not just in the summer. Adding herbs to a dish is one of the easiest and most affordable ways to increase both the nutrients and the flavour. Tending your own herb garden is incredibly relaxing and helps you live in the present moment. These burgers are truly a reflection of what was bursting with life in my herb garden that day! The result was incredibly tasty meat-free, plant-based burgers that are packed with protein.

My favourite brand of tempeh is Henry's Tempeh because it's both organic and gluten-free. If you don't have fresh herbs, use dried herbs, but use a much smaller amount. I would suggest 1 tablespoon (15 mL) each of dried parsley and basil and 1 teaspoon (5 mL) dried dill. Enjoy with my Crunchy Beet and Carrot Quinoa Salad (page 103).

1 package (8 ounces/225 g) organic tempeh
2 tablespoons (30 mL) extra-virgin olive oil
1 small red onion, chopped
3 cloves garlic, chopped
¾ cup (175 mL) chopped cremini mushrooms
½ cup (125 mL) almond flour (almond meal)
½ cup (125 mL) loosely packed chopped fresh curly parsley
½ cup (125 mL) loosely packed chopped fresh basil
¼ cup (60 mL) loosely packed chopped fresh dill
½ teaspoon (2 mL) sea salt
½ teaspoon (2 mL) pepper
1 egg
2 tablespoons (30 mL) coconut oil

For serving
4 gluten-free whole-grain burger buns
Spinach Walnut Pesto (page 192)
Quick Pickled Onions (page 133)
Sliced dill pickles
Sliced tomatoes
Sliced avocado

1. Preheat the oven to 375°F (190°C). Line a baking sheet with parchment paper.

2. Slice the tempeh into chunks and pulse in a food processor until crumbly. Leave it in the food processor.

3. Heat the olive oil in a medium frying pan over medium heat. Add the red onion, garlic and mushrooms and cook, stirring frequently, until the onions are soft and translucent, about 5 minutes. Transfer the mixture to the food processor.

4. Add the almond flour, parsley, basil, dill, sea salt, pepper and egg. Pulse until combined. Shape the mixture into 4 patties, each about 1 inch (2.5 cm) thick.

5. Wipe the frying pan clean, then melt the coconut oil over medium heat. Place the patties in the pan and cook until golden brown, 5 to 6 minutes per side. Transfer the patties to the prepared baking sheet and bake for 20 minutes, turning halfway through.

6. Place the burgers on burger buns and spread with Spinach Walnut Pesto. Top with Quick Pickled Onions, dill pickles, tomato and avocado.

Super-Quick Tuna Burgers
Dairy-free • Gluten-free • Grain-free • Kid-friendly

Serves 4 to 6

These bunless burgers are so full of flavour you won't miss your favourite beef burger for a second. True to the name, these are burgers you can whip up super quickly with ingredients you probably already have in your kitchen. Of course you can use fresh tuna steaks if you're feeling fancy, but I always keep a few cans of white tuna packed in water in my pantry for just these kind of quickie recipes. The combination of tamari, sesame, ginger and cilantro gives these burgers a delectable Asian flavour you won't soon forget.

Enjoy these burgers in summer with a nice big mixed green salad like my Summer Salad with Halloumi (page 96). If you're serving the burgers in the winter, enjoy them with my Baked Cauliflower and Broccoli with Tahini Lemon Sauce (page 112).

2 cans (5½ ounces/150 g each) water-
    packed solid white tuna, drained
1 cup (250 mL) almond flour (almond
    meal)
1 tablespoon (15 mL) garlic powder
2 eggs, whisked
½ cup (125 mL) loosely packed chopped
    fresh cilantro
⅓ cup (75 mL) chopped green onion
    (white and light green parts only)
2 tablespoons (30 mL) gluten-free tamari
2 tablespoons (30 mL) toasted sesame oil
1 teaspoon (5 mL) grated fresh ginger
1 tablespoon (15 mL) extra-virgin olive
    oil or coconut oil
Creamy Tahini Dressing (page 107),
    for serving

1. In a large bowl, mix together the tuna, almond flour and garlic powder. Add the whisked eggs, cilantro, green onions, tamari, sesame oil and ginger.

2. Mix well and shape the mixture into 6 patties, each about ¾ inch (2 cm) thick. If you prefer larger burgers, form the mixture into 4 patties.

3. In a large frying pan, heat the olive oil over medium heat. Add the patties and cook until golden brown and crispy, 5 to 7 minutes per side. Be careful not to burn them. Serve the burgers topped with Creamy Tahini Dressing.

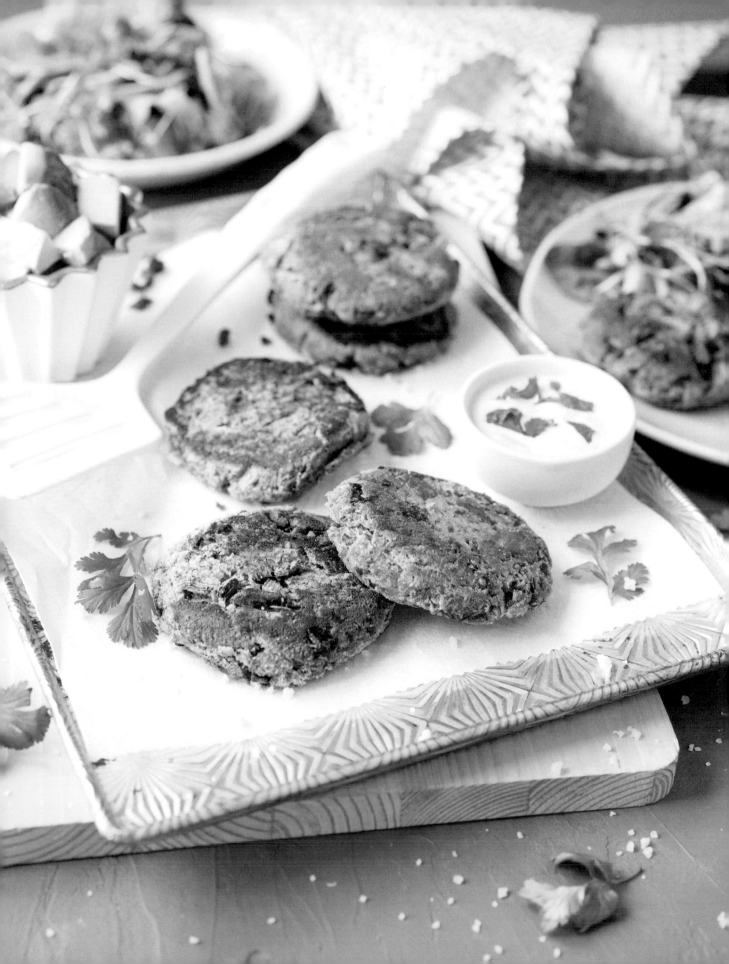

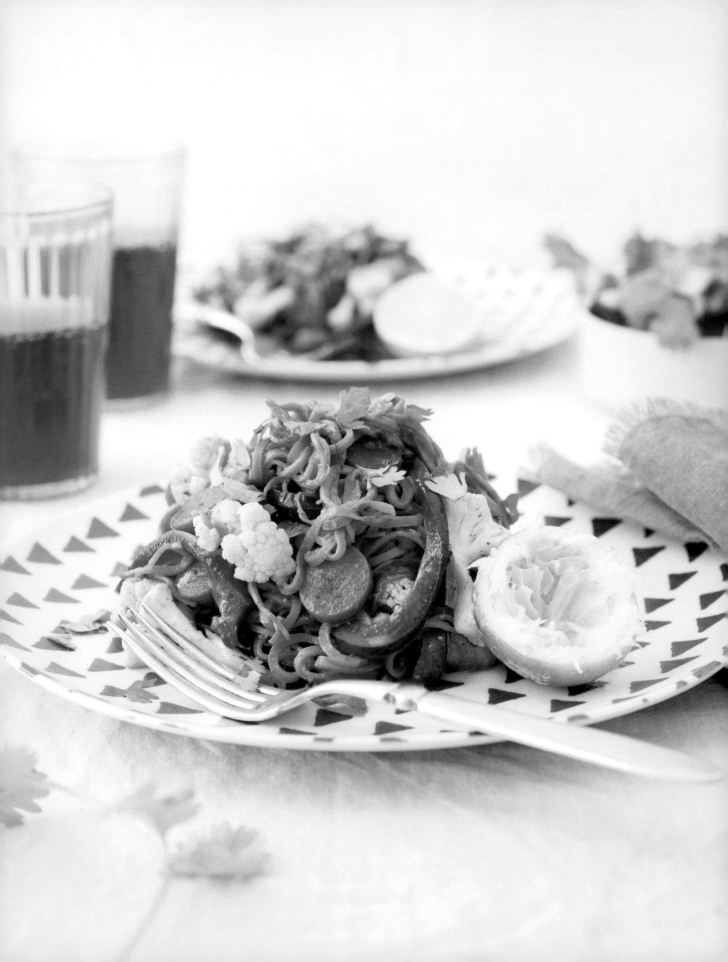

Sweet Potato Veggie Pad Thai

Dairy-free • Gluten-free • Grain-free • Vegan

Serves 2

My colleague and friend Rachel loves Thai food and has taken cooking classes in Thailand. She adds a Thai flavour to almost everything she cooks. She told Walker and me that her pad Thai was epic, so we put her to the test and she made it for us. We were hooked! Since then we have made it countless times. I love that this recipe contains no refined sugar and the noodles are delicious spiralized sweet potato.

This recipe serves two generously, but if you're doubling it to serve four people, I recommend cooking it in two separate batches because it's too much for one pan. Enjoy this dish with my Veggie Rolls with Spicy Almond Sauce (page 125).

Sauce

¼ cup (60 mL) extra-virgin olive oil
¼ cup (60 mL) gluten-free tamari
¼ cup (60 mL) natural smooth almond butter
2 tablespoons (30 mL) real maple syrup
1 to 2 teaspoons (5 to 10 mL) red chili flakes
Juice of ½ lime
2 cloves garlic, minced
1-inch (2.5 cm) piece of fresh ginger, peeled and minced
Sea salt

Sweet Potato Veggie Pad Thai

1 to 2 tablespoons (15 to 30 mL) extra-virgin olive oil
2 cups (500 mL) carrots cut into ¼-inch (5 mm) rounds
2 cups (500 mL) cauliflower florets
1 small sweet red pepper, cut into matchsticks
1 large sweet potato, peeled and spiralized
2 tablespoons (30 mL) fresh cilantro leaves, for garnish

1. **Make the Sauce** In a small bowl, whisk together the olive oil, tamari, almond butter, maple syrup, chili flakes, lime juice, garlic, ginger and sea salt to taste. Set aside.

2. **Make the Sweet Potato Veggie Pad Thai** Heat the olive oil in a large frying pan over medium heat. Add the carrots and cauliflower and cook, stirring occasionally, for 10 minutes, or until tender. Add the red pepper and cook for another 2 to 3 minutes. Transfer to a large bowl.

3. Return the pan (you don't need to wipe it clean) to medium heat. Drizzle the pan with a bit more olive oil and add the spiralized sweet potato. Cook for 6 to 7 minutes, just until the potatoes look a bit glossy. Be careful you don't overcook them.

4. Scrape the sweet potato into the bowl with the other vegetables and pour the reserved sauce over top. Mix with tongs to ensure the sauce covers everything. Divide evenly between 2 plates and garnish with cilantro.

Mushroom Falafel Balls

Dairy-free • Kid-friendly • Nut-free • Vegan

Makes 32 falafels, serves 4 to 6

These falafel balls are the perfect texture—crunchy on the outside and soft on the inside. Packed with fibre and flavour, these balls make a wonderful lunch or dinner. When I want a grain-free meal I forgo the pita and mix the falafels into a big salad. Either way, whip up a batch of my Creamy Tahini Dressing to drizzle over the falafel balls.

If you want perfectly shaped falafel balls, use a cookie-dough scoop. You can also flatten the balls into patties. Enjoy my Dark Chocolate Superfood Bars (page 224) for dessert and you've got the perfect plant-based meal from start to finish.

1 tablespoon (15 mL) extra-virgin olive oil or coconut oil

1 small white onion, chopped

2 cloves garlic, chopped

1½ cups (375 mL) sliced cremini or white button mushrooms

1 can (14 ounces/398 mL) chickpeas, drained and rinsed

1 cup (250 mL) brown rice flour

½ cup (125 mL) loosely packed chopped fresh curly or flat-leaf parsley

½ cup (125 mL) loosely packed chopped fresh cilantro

1 tablespoon (15 mL) ground cumin

½ teaspoon (2 mL) sea salt

¼ to ½ teaspoon (1 to 2 mL) cayenne pepper

Juice of ½ lemon

For serving

Shredded lettuce

Raw vegetables such as carrot matchsticks, sliced radish, shredded purple cabbage

6 small gluten-free or whole wheat pitas

½ cup (125 mL) Creamy Tahini Dressing (page 107)

1. Preheat the oven to 375°F (190°C). Line a baking sheet with parchment paper or grease with coconut oil.

2. Heat the olive oil in a large frying pan over medium heat. Add the onion and garlic and cook, stirring occasionally, until the onions are soft and translucent, 4 to 5 minutes. Add the mushrooms and cook until fork-tender, about 5 minutes. Remove from the heat.

3. In a food processor, combine the chickpeas, brown rice flour, parsley, cilantro, cumin, sea salt, cayenne and lemon juice. Pulse until well blended. Add the mushroom mixture and pulse again until blended.

4. Using about 1½ tablespoons (22 mL) of the mixture at a time, roll between your hands into balls. (If making patties, flatten the balls into ½-inch/1 cm discs.) Place the falafel balls on the prepared baking sheet and bake for 15 minutes, until golden brown on the bottom. Turn the balls and bake for another 15 to 20 minutes, until golden brown all over.

5. To serve, place vegetables of your choice on top of a pita, top with 4 or 5 falafel balls and drizzle with the Creamy Tahini Dressing. Store any leftovers in an airtight container in the fridge for up to 5 days.

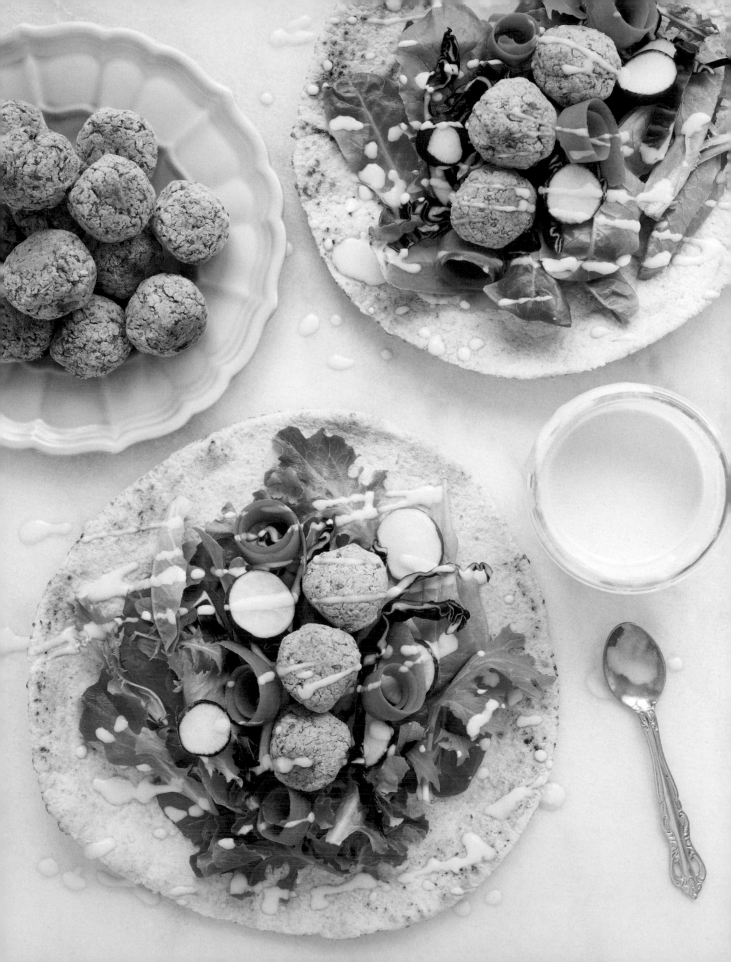

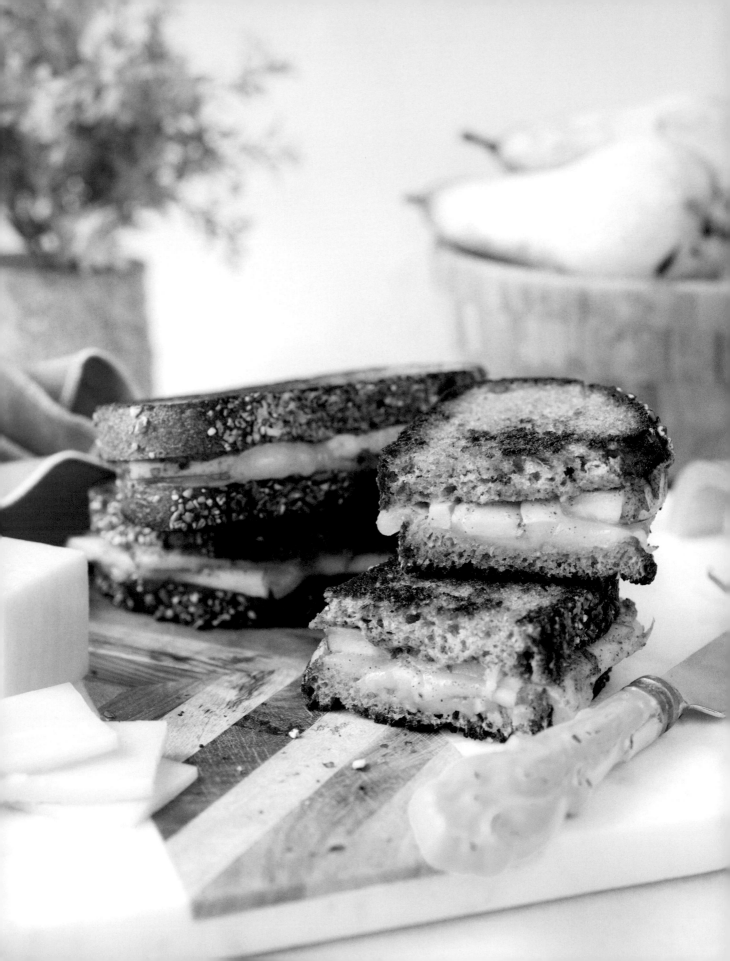

Grilled Cheese and Pear Sammies

Kid-friendly • Nut-free • Vegetarian

Makes 4 sandwiches

This is my healthy take on a Canadian classic that is typically made with processed cheese. When I was a kid the only time I ate grilled cheese sandwiches made with processed cheese singles was when I had lunch at my babysitter's house. At home my mom made grilled cheese sammies with real cheese—the way they should be made! The cheese melted properly and didn't make my stomach feel like it was turned inside out, and the sandwich tasted oh so good! Here I have added pear and Dijon mustard to make this sandwich soar to new heights.

If you don't have pears on hand, then try this with apple. Enjoy with my Roasted Red Pepper Soup (page 148).

8 slices of sourdough bread

2 tablespoons (30 mL) unsalted butter, Turmeric Ghee (page 43) or store-bought ghee

4 teaspoons (20 mL) Dijon mustard

1½ cups (375 mL) grated white cheddar cheese

2 ripe firm Bosc or Bartlett pears, cored and thinly sliced

1. Heat a grill pan or large frying pan over medium heat. If your frying pan isn't large enough to hold all 4 sandwiches, use 2 pans or cook them in batches.

2. Spread the butter on one side of each slice of bread and spread the mustard on the other side. Place 4 slices of bread buttered side down in the pan. Divide the cheese and pear evenly among the slices. Just when the cheese is starting to melt, top the sandwiches with the remaining bread, buttered side up, and cook until golden brown on the bottom, 2 to 3 minutes. Flip and continue to cook for 1 to 2 minutes, until golden brown on the bottom.

Fish Tacos with Tomato Cilantro Salsa

Dairy-free • Kid-friendly • Nut-free

Makes 4 tacos

Tacos are the ultimate summer food—fresh, bright, flavourful. This is one of my favourite recipes for entertaining in the summer because it's easy and always a winner. I make the salsa a few hours ahead so the flavours can mingle, and the fish requires very little prep. This means I can socialize more! These tacos go nicely with my Peach and Snap Pea Salad (page 99) followed by Strawberries and Cream Freezer Fudge (page 239) for a complete and healthy meal.

You could also grill the fish on the barbecue for 10 to 15 minutes. Be sure to wrap the fish in foil before placing it on the barbecue so it doesn't fall apart.

Taco Filling

4 skinless halibut or sole fillets
  (2 to 3 ounces/55 to 85 g each)
Sea salt and pepper

Tomato Cilantro Salsa

1 cup (250 mL) grape tomatoes, quartered
¼ cup (60 mL) loosely packed chopped
  fresh cilantro
¼ red onion, finely chopped
3 green onions (white and light green
  parts only), chopped
Sea salt

For assembly

4 large soft taco shells or tortillas
¼ cup (60 mL) loosely packed chopped
  fresh cilantro
Juice of 1 lime

1. **Make the Taco Filling** Preheat the oven to 375°F (190°C). Line a baking sheet with parchment paper.

2. Place the fish on the baking sheet. Sprinkle with a pinch each of sea salt and pepper. Bake for 15 to 20 minutes, until the fish flakes easily with a fork.

3. Flake the fish with a fork and leave it on the baking sheet until you are ready to assemble the tacos.

4. **Meanwhile, make the Tomato Cilantro Salsa** In a small bowl, combine the tomatoes, cilantro, red onion, green onions and a pinch of sea salt.

5. **Assemble the tacos** Place a quarter of the flaked fish in each taco shell or tortilla. Top with the Tomato Cilantro Salsa and garnish with fresh cilantro and a drizzle of lime juice.

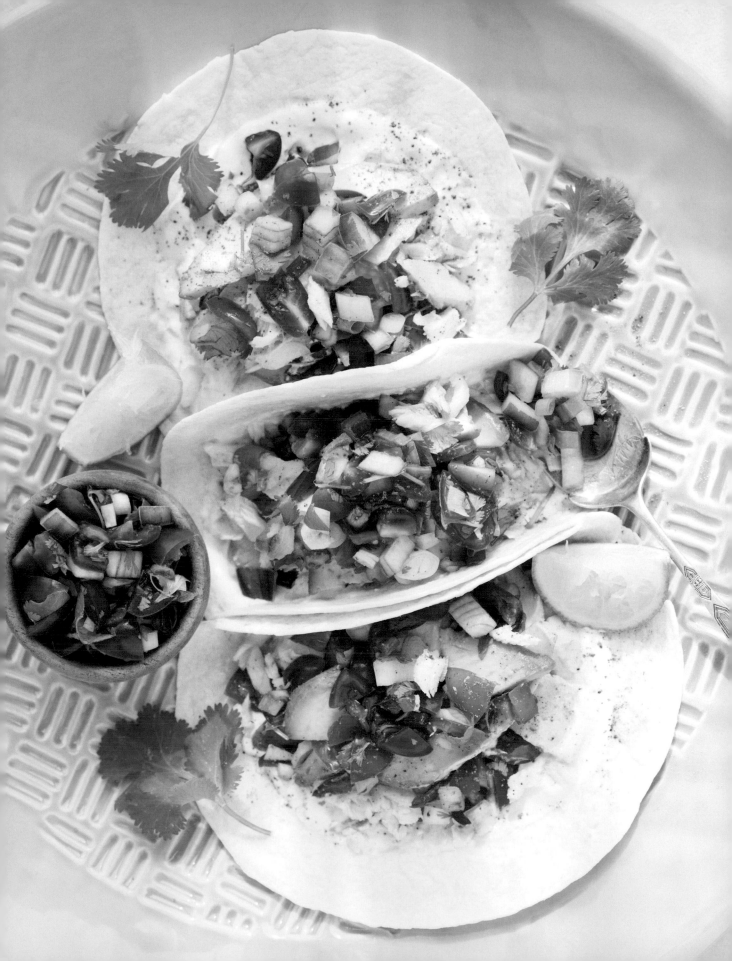

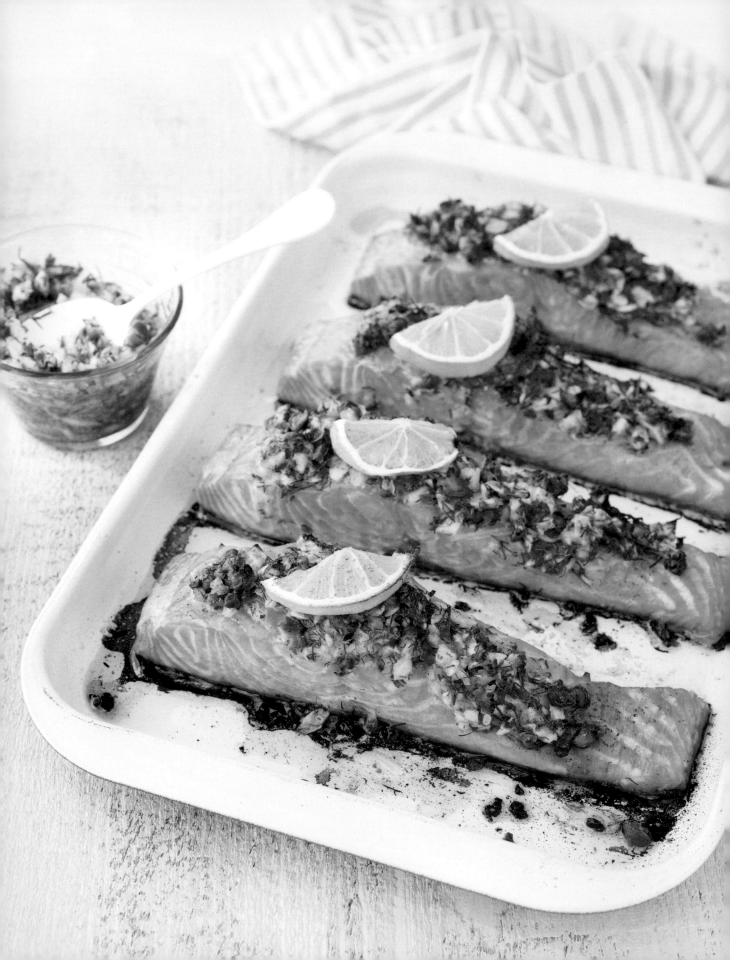

Baked Salmon with Caper Dill Pesto

Dairy-free • Gluten-free • Grain-free • Kid-friendly • Nut-free

Serves 4

This recipe is from my good friend Shelby. She is an amazing cook, one of those people who never follows a recipe but whose dishes always turn out incredible. When she told me she had this awesome caper pesto, I had to try it. And being Shelby's, it's absolutely delicious! The combination of salty capers with herbaceous dill is a memorable match. This pesto makes salmon—or any fish, for that matter—soar to new heights.

Salmon is an excellent source of omega-3 fatty acids, which are important for heart health, and vitamin D for a healthy immune system. If you're making this dish in the warmer months, I recommend serving it with my Chilled Zucchini Avocado Basil Soup (page 139). Finish it off with the Blackberry and Strawberry Galette (page 216) and you've got an evening to remember.

Caper Dill Pesto

1 small white onion, roughly chopped
1 to 2 cloves garlic
½ cup (125 mL) loosely packed fresh dill
¼ cup (60 mL) drained capers
3 tablespoons (45 mL) extra-virgin olive oil
½ teaspoon (2 mL) red chili flakes
Black pepper

Baked Salmon

4 wild or organic farmed salmon fillets
   (3 to 4 ounces/85 to 115 g each)
Sea salt and freshly ground pepper
Juice of 1 lemon
Fresh dill sprigs, for garnish
Lemon wedges, for garnish

1. Preheat the oven to 375°F (190°C). Line a baking sheet with parchment paper.

2. Make the Caper Dill Pesto In a small food processor, combine the onion, garlic, dill, capers, olive oil and chili flakes. Pulse until coarsely chopped. Season with black pepper.

3. Make the Baked Salmon Place the fish on the prepared baking sheet. Season with sea salt and pepper. Spread the Caper Dill Pesto over the fillets. Bake for 15 to 20 minutes, until the fish flakes easily with a fork.

4. Arrange the fillets on plates, drizzle with lemon juice, top with dill and garnish with a lemon wedge on the side. Serve immediately.

Spinach Walnut Pesto Pasta Bowl

Gluten-free • Kid-friendly • Vegetarian

Serves 4

This pasta dish has my daughter Vienna's name written all over it. She has always preferred a pesto to a marinara sauce for pasta (just like her mama), and this pasta bowl is loaded up with all her favourite veggies. It's flavourful and filling, especially if you use chickpea pasta, so it makes my belly joyous too. I don't bother cooking the veggies—I just mix everything together while the pasta is warm, so everything stays nice and crunchy. Sometimes I chill it and serve it as a salad. However it's served, when we are finished you'd think someone had licked the bowl!

This recipe makes a big batch of spinach pesto, so you may have leftovers for other dishes, like my Super-Quick Tortilla Pizzas (page 175). My Almond Butter Rice Crispy Squares (page 220) are the perfect dessert for this kid-friendly meal.

8 ounces (225 g) quinoa pasta or chickpea pasta
1 sweet yellow pepper, chopped
1 cup (250 mL) fresh or thawed frozen peas
1 cup (250 mL) grape or cherry tomatoes, cut in half
½ cup (125 mL) finely chopped red onion or green onion (white and light green parts only)
Grated Parmesan cheese or nutritional yeast, for serving
Fresh basil leaves, for garnish

Spinach Walnut Pesto
2 cups (500 mL) tightly packed fresh baby spinach
½ cup (125 mL) loosely packed fresh basil leaves
¾ cup (175 mL) raw walnuts
¼ cup (60 mL) extra-virgin olive oil
2 tablespoons (30 mL) lemon juice
Sea salt

1. Bring a large pot of water to a boil. Add the pasta and cook according to package instructions or until desired tenderness.

2. Meanwhile, in a large serving bowl, combine the yellow pepper, peas, tomatoes and red onion. Set aside.

3. **Make the Spinach Walnut Pesto** Combine the spinach, basil, walnuts, olive oil and lemon juice in a food processor. Blend until smooth. Season with sea salt.

4. Add the drained pasta to the bowl of vegetables. Add as much Spinach Walnut Pesto as you want and mix together. Add a drizzle of olive oil if the pasta looks dry. Sprinkle with Parmesan, garnish with basil leaves and serve immediately. Store any leftover pesto in an airtight container in the fridge for up to 2 days.

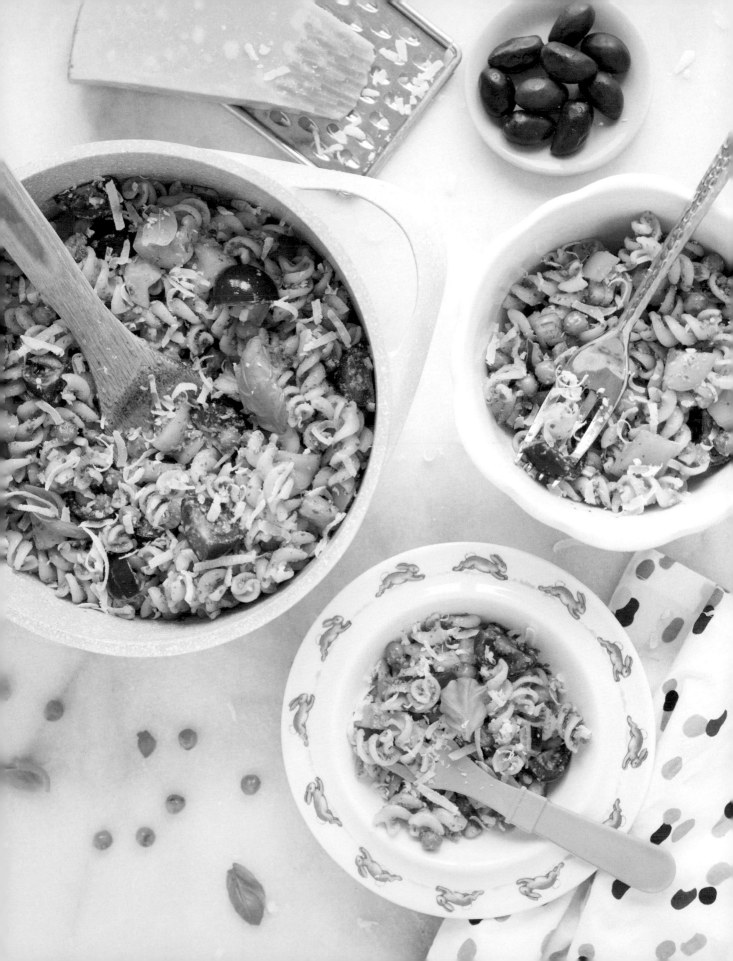

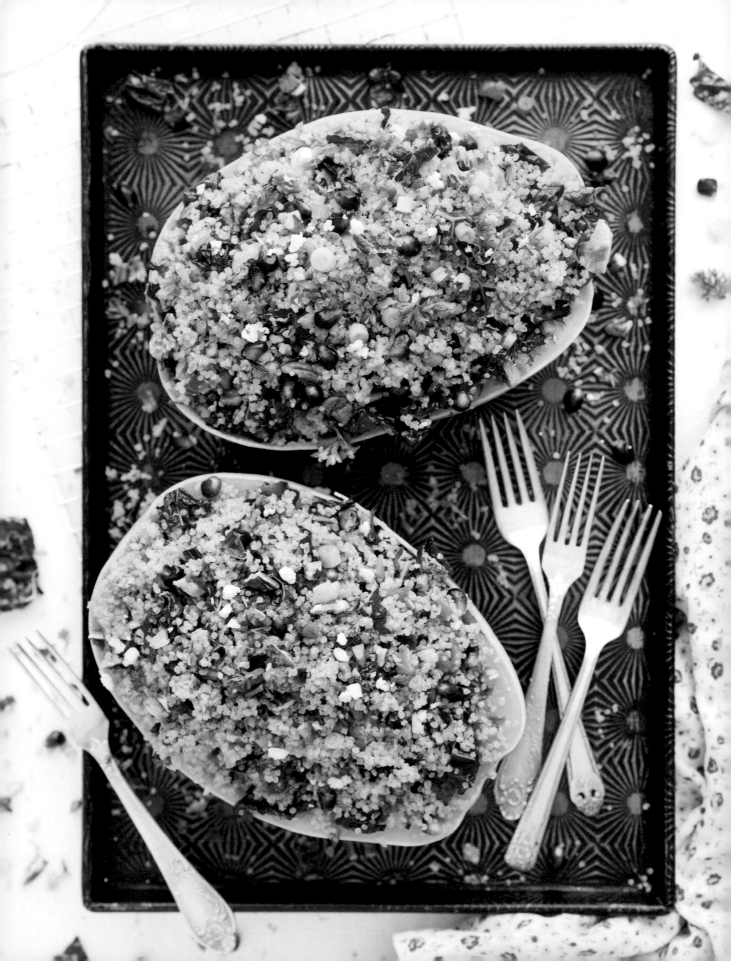

Quinoa-Stuffed Spaghetti Squash

Gluten-free · Kid-friendly · Vegetarian

Serves 2 to 4

I love making this dish on crisp autumn nights because it's hearty and warming to the core. Adding the pomegranate seeds together with the quinoa lends the perfect variety of textures, plus a burst of flavour and juice. For perfect timing, once you've cooked the squash about halfway, make the stuffing. That way it's nice and hot when you put it into the squash and you don't have to reheat it. If you have leftover stuffing, consider yourself lucky—you've got lunch for tomorrow! This recipe can be the main for two people or a side for four people. When I make this for four people, I usually cut a larger squash in half width-wise once it's cooked. If you're making this for a toddler, scrape out the spaghetti squash and serve it alongside the stuffing, just to make it easier for little hands. If you're feeding a baby, you could put all the ingredients into a food processor and give it a blitz to make a purée.

My hubs, Walker, is always super helpful in the kitchen, so if I'm making this, he's usually whipping up a healthy side to go with it like a big salad or my Garlicky Green Beans with Tahini Lemon Sauce (page 118).

1 large or 2 small spaghetti squash, cut in half lengthwise and seeds removed

1½ cups (375 mL) white quinoa

3 cups (750 mL) water

1 tablespoon (15 mL) coconut oil

½ large red onion, finely chopped

1 bunch lacinato kale, centre stems removed, chopped into bite-size pieces

½ cup (125 mL) pomegranate seeds

½ cup (125 mL) loosely packed chopped fresh curly parsley

¼ cup (60 mL) chopped green onions (white and light green parts only)

¼ cup (60 mL) chopped raw pecans

½ teaspoon (2 mL) cinnamon

¼ teaspoon (1 mL) ground allspice

1 tablespoon (15 mL) extra-virgin olive oil

Sea salt and pepper

¼ cup (60 mL) crumbled feta cheese (optional)

1. Preheat the oven to 400°F (200°C). Line a baking sheet with parchment paper.

2. Place the squash on the prepared baking sheet with the flesh side down. Add a touch of water to the pan so the squash doesn't dry out. Bake for 45 to 50 minutes, until the squash is fork-tender and you can easily scrape the flesh away from the skin with a fork. Be careful not to overcook the squash—you don't want it soggy.

3. Meanwhile, in a medium saucepan, combine the quinoa and water. Bring to a gentle boil, then reduce the heat and simmer, with the lid slightly ajar, for 15 minutes, or until fluffy. Transfer the quinoa to a large bowl. Cover to keep warm.

4. While the quinoa cooks, melt the coconut oil in a large frying pan over medium heat. Add the red onion and cook, stirring frequently, until soft and translucent, 4 to 5 minutes. Add the kale and cook for 1 to 2 minutes. Add the mixture to the quinoa along with the pomegranate seeds, parsley, green onions, pecans, cinnamon and allspice. Stir well. Drizzle with olive oil and season with sea salt and pepper. Cover to keep warm.

5. Remove the squash from the oven and scoop the warm quinoa stuffing into each half. Top with feta (if using) and serve immediately.

Zucchini Noodles with Turkey Meatballs

Dairy-free • Gluten-free • Grain-free • Kid-friendly

Makes 24 meatballs, serves 4 to 6

These turkey meatballs are a hit in my home every time I make them. Sometimes I serve them as a side dish, without zucchini noodles or sauce, with a big salad and roasted veggies. They are also a crowd-pleaser for entertaining. Just stick a toothpick in each one and serve as hors d'oeuvres. But trust me, it's worth the extra effort to make my Homemade Tomato Sauce and spiralize zucchini for a whole and complete meal! I love using zucchini instead of grain-based noodles for pasta because it's much lighter and it's fun to change it up. Plus, it's a great way to get kids to eat more veggies.

   If using plain tomato sauce, add dried herbs such as 1 teaspoon (5 mL) crumbled dried rosemary, 1 teaspoon (5 mL) dried basil or parsley, and 1 minced garlic clove to the sauce for flavour.

1 pound (450 g) ground organic turkey or chicken

½ medium white onion, finely chopped

2 to 3 cloves garlic, finely chopped

½ cup (125 mL) almond flour (almond meal)

¼ cup (60 mL) loosely packed chopped fresh curly parsley

¼ cup (60 mL) loosely packed chopped fresh basil

2 tablespoons (30 mL) gluten-free tamari

2 tablespoons (30 mL) Dijon mustard

6 cups (1.5 L) Homemade Tomato Sauce (page 156) or store-bought

1 tablespoon (15 mL) extra-virgin olive oil, more for serving

4 zucchini, spiralized or peeled using a vegetable peeler

Chopped fresh basil or flat-leaf parsley, for garnish

1. Preheat the oven to 350°F (180°C). Line a baking sheet with parchment paper.

2. In a large bowl, combine the turkey, onion, garlic, almond flour, parsley, basil, tamari and mustard. Mix well. Using about 1½ tablespoons (22 mL) of the mixture at a time, roll between your hands into 1½-inch (4 cm) balls. Arrange the meatballs on the prepared baking sheet.

3. Bake for 15 minutes, or until brown on the bottom. Turn and cook for another 10 to 15 minutes, until brown and cooked through.

4. Meanwhile, in a large pot, heat the Homemade Tomato Sauce over medium heat. Add the meatballs to the sauce. (The meatballs and sauce can be set aside at this point. Reheat before serving.)

5. Heat the olive oil in a large frying pan over medium heat. Add the zucchini noodles and cook, tossing gently, until just until warmed. Spoon the zucchini noodles into the tomato sauce and stir to combine. (You can skip this step and just add the uncooked zucchini noodles to the tomato sauce.) Serve topped with basil and drizzle with olive oil.

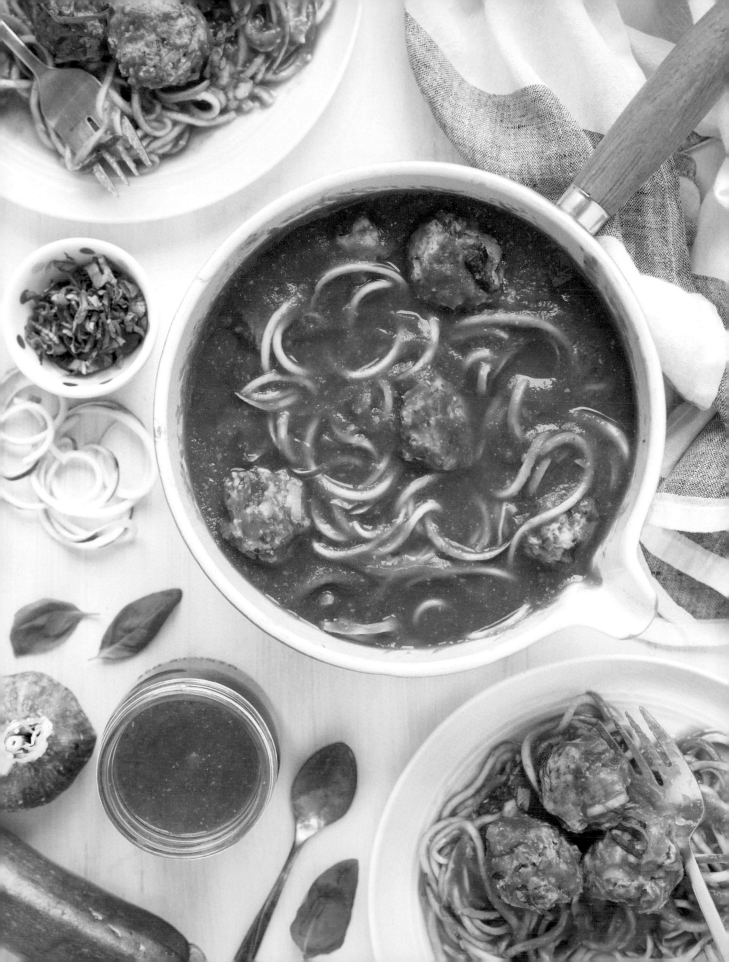

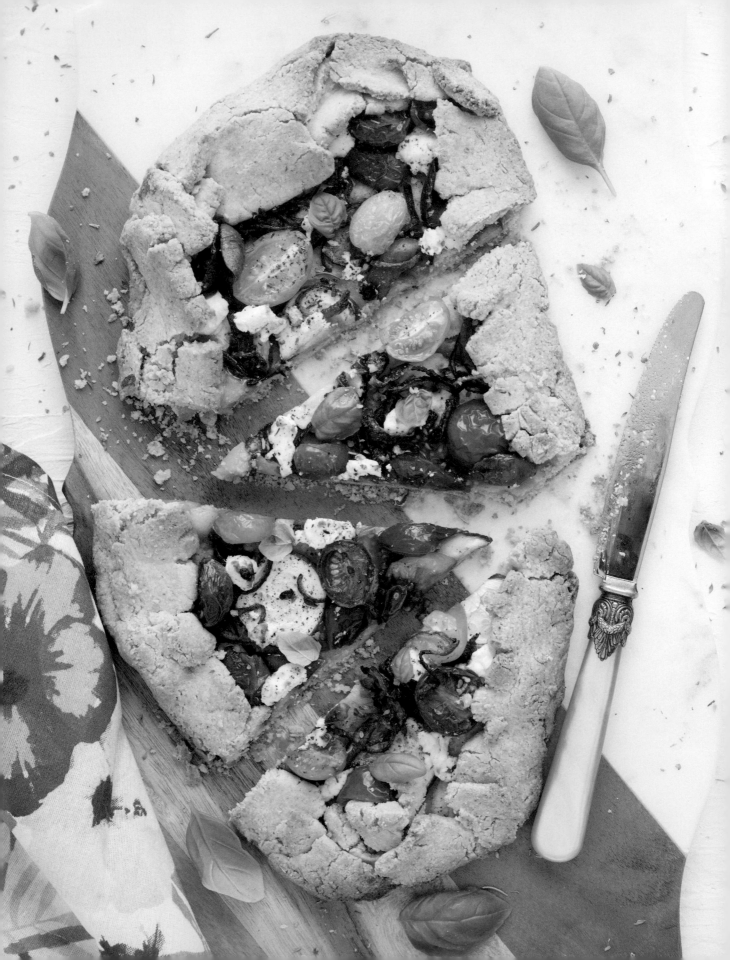

Rustic Mediterranean Summer Galette

Gluten-free · Grain-free · Kid-friendly · Vegetarian

Serves 4 to 6

A galette sounds kind of fancy but it's just the French word for a free-form tart. They are much easier to make than a pie or a torte, and I'm totally addicted to making both savoury and sweet galettes.

This galette screams *Mediterranean summer* with fresh basil, local tomatoes and zucchini. The crust is totally gluten-free, which surprises most people because it has such a wonderful texture. It's also quite filling, because the main ingredient in the crust is almond flour, which is full of good fat and protein. So even though it doesn't seem like much to serve four people, if you serve this with a big salad, you've got a satisfying dinner for four.

Crust

1½ cups (375 mL) almond flour
  (almond meal)
½ cup (125 mL) tapioca starch/flour
1 tablespoon (15 mL) dried rosemary
1 teaspoon (5 mL) garlic powder
½ teaspoon (2 mL) sea salt
6 tablespoons (90 mL) cold unsalted
  butter, cubed
2 eggs, divided

Filling

1 tablespoon (15 mL) extra-virgin olive oil
1 small red onion, thinly sliced
1 small zucchini, sliced into rounds
6 grape tomatoes, cut in half
5 or 6 pitted green olives, cut in half
3 to 4 tablespoons (45 to 60 mL) crumbled
  goat cheese
Sea salt and pepper
Fresh basil leaves, for garnish

1. **Make the Crust** In a food processor, combine the almond flour, tapioca starch, rosemary, garlic powder, sea salt and butter. Pulse until the mixture is the texture of coarse meal.

2. Add 1 egg and pulse just until the dough comes together in small chunks. Scrape the dough out onto a work surface and shape into a ball. Flatten into a 5-inch (12 cm) disc, wrap with plastic wrap and chill in the fridge for at least 1 hour or in the freezer for 30 minutes.

3. **Meanwhile, prepare the Filling** Heat the olive oil in a medium frying pan over medium heat. Add the red onion and cook, stirring occasionally, until the onions are soft, 4 to 5 minutes. Add the zucchini and cook, stirring occasionally, for another 5 minutes, or until the zucchini is soft. Remove from the heat and let cool.

4. Preheat the oven to 375°F (190°C).

5. **Assemble the Galette** On a floured sheet of parchment paper and using a rolling pin sprinkled with flour, roll out the dough into a 10-inch (25 cm) circle. It's okay if it's not perfectly shaped. Slide the pastry, on the parchment paper, onto a baking sheet.

6. Spread the filling in the centre of the dough, stopping 2 to 2½ inches (5 to 6 cm) from the edge. Scatter the tomatoes, olives and goat cheese evenly over the filling. Fold the dough border up over the sides, overlapping in pleats here and there. Don't worry if the dough cracks as you fold it. Just press the dough with your fingers to seal the crack. It doesn't have to look perfect.

7. In a small bowl, whisk the remaining egg. Brush the folded-over dough with the egg wash for a golden top edge. Sprinkle the galette with sea salt and pepper to taste. Bake for 35 minutes, or until the crust is golden brown. Let stand for 5 minutes, then garnish with basil, slice and serve. Store in an airtight container in the fridge for up to 5 days.

Lamb Chops with Orange Mint Marmalade

Dairy-free • Gluten-free • Grain-free • Kid-friendly • Nut-free

Serves 4

My friend in high school was Welsh and he grew up eating lamb like it was his job. So of course my introduction to lamb was dinner at his house, made by his mother. I still remember how she made it, the traditional way, roasted and served with mint sauce. I fell in love with lamb and I have been hooked ever since. Instead of roasting it, I brown marinated chops in a grill pan, which is a lot easier and faster than roasting a whole leg!

Instead of mint sauce I've combined fresh mint with a hit of citrus. I love this combination—it's a feast for your taste buds! To speed things up, you can make the Orange Mint Marmalade in a mini food processor. We enjoy this with my Sticky Turmeric Paprika Carrots (page 115) or Roasted Root Veggies (page 116) for a nourishing and flavourful meal.

Zest and juice of 2 large oranges
¼ cup (60 mL) loosely packed finely chopped fresh curly or flat-leaf parsley
3 cloves garlic, minced
¼ cup (60 mL) + 2 tablespoons (30 mL) extra-virgin olive oil, divided
8 lamb rib chops
½ teaspoon (2 mL) sea salt
Pinch of pepper

Orange Mint Marmalade
Peel of 1 orange, finely chopped
¼ cup (60 mL) loosely packed finely chopped fresh mint
3 tablespoons (45 mL) pure liquid honey

1. **Marinate the Lamb Chops** In a small bowl, whisk together the orange zest, orange juice, parsley, garlic and ¼ cup (60 mL) of the olive oil.

2. Place the lamb chops in a shallow baking dish large enough to hold them snugly. Pour the marinade over the lamb chops and season with the sea salt and pepper. Let sit in the fridge for 1 to 2 hours.

3. **Make the Orange Mint Marmalade** In a small bowl, stir together the orange peel, mint and honey.

4. In a grill pan, heat the remaining 2 tablespoons (30 mL) olive oil over medium heat. Brown the lamb chops for about 5 minutes per side or until desired doneness. Serve immediately, topped with the Orange Mint Marmalade.

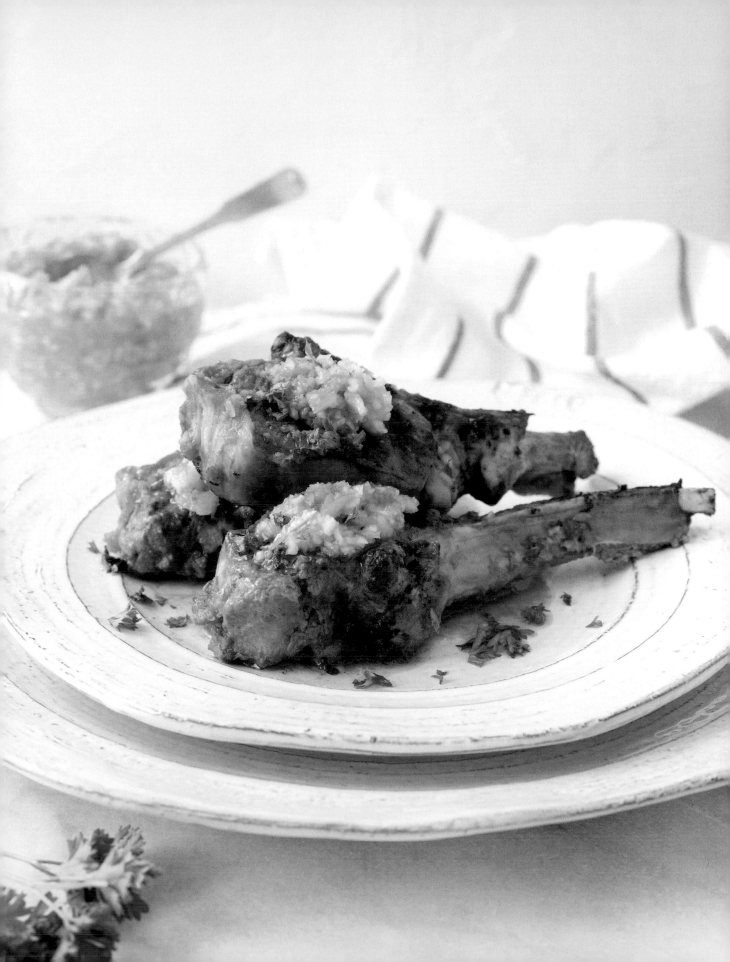

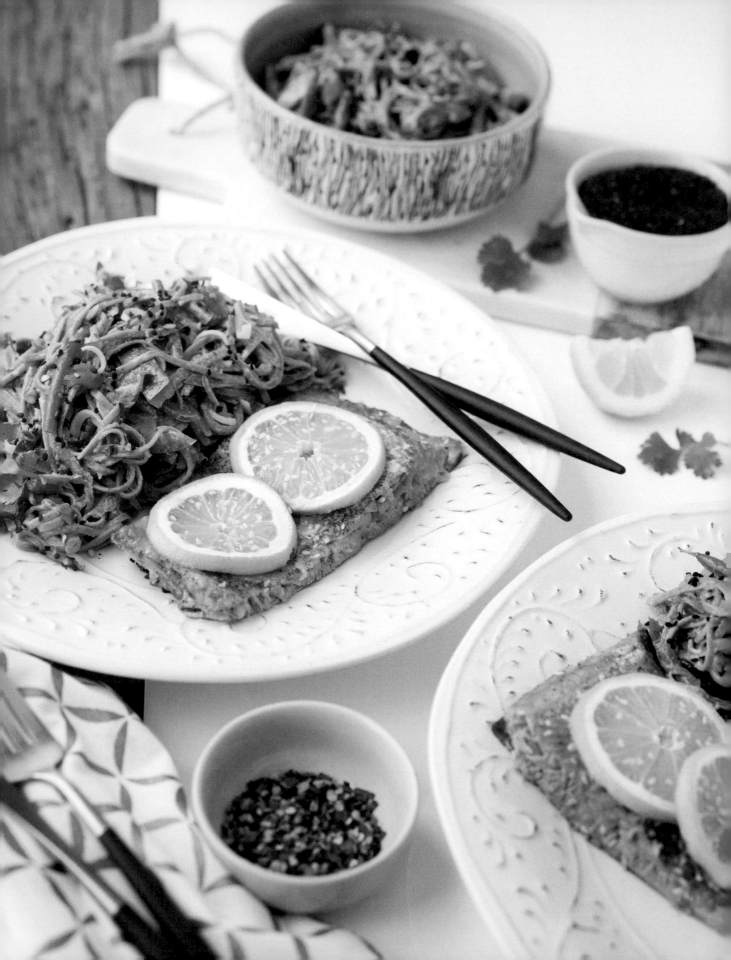

Lemon Pepper Baked Trout

Gluten-free • Grain-free • Kid-friendly • Nut-free

Serves 4

We eat fish a couple of times a week because it's such a nourishing food. It's a great source of good fats, complete protein and minerals such as iron, zinc, magnesium, potassium and B vitamins. It helps that my daughter loves it too. We started feeding Vienna fish before she turned one.

The secret to delicious fish is not overcooking it. This recipe is so juicy and versatile that we use it with trout, arctic char or salmon. This fish goes well with my Crunchy and Creamy Soba Noodle Salad with Almond Dressing (page 111). For dessert, the Coconut Black Rice Pudding (page 215) is a perfect match.

4 trout fillets (4 ounces/115 g each)
½ teaspoon (2 mL) garlic powder
¼ teaspoon (1 mL) dried basil or parsley
Pinch each of sea salt and pepper
2 tablespoons (30 mL) Italian-Seasoned Ghee (page 44), store-bought ghee or unsalted butter
Juice of 1 lemon
8 lemon wedges

1. Preheat the oven to 375°F (190°C). Line a baking sheet with parchment paper.

2. Place the fillets skin side down on the prepared baking sheet. Sprinkle with the garlic powder, dried basil, sea salt and pepper. Spread the Italian-Seasoned Ghee on top of the fillets. Sprinkle with lemon juice and place 2 lemon wedges on each fillet. Bake for 15 minutes, or until the fish is cooked through.

Paprika Barbecue Sauce

Dairy-free • Gluten-free • Grain-free • Kid-friendly • Nut-free • Vegan

Makes about 1 cup (250 mL)

Once I started making my own barbecue sauce, I never wanted to buy it again. It is super easy to make and you will avoid the excessive amounts of salt and sugar found in store-bought varieties. I change this up depending on what I will be doing with it. I love honey garlic sauce, so instead of maple syrup and garlic powder I use honey and fresh or roasted garlic. This barbecue sauce is the perfect dipping sauce for my Crispy Chicken Fingers (page 176) or to slather on Herby Tempeh Burgers (page 179). If you have time, make this ahead and refrigerate overnight to let the flavours mingle.

2 cans (5½ ounces/156 mL each) tomato paste
½ cup (125 mL) real maple syrup
½ cup (125 mL) gluten-free tamari
2 teaspoons (10 mL) garlic powder
1 teaspoon (5 mL) sweet paprika
¼ teaspoon (1 mL) cayenne pepper
1 teaspoon (5 mL) apple cider vinegar (optional)

1. In a small bowl, whisk together all the ingredients. Store in an airtight container in the fridge for up to 2 weeks.

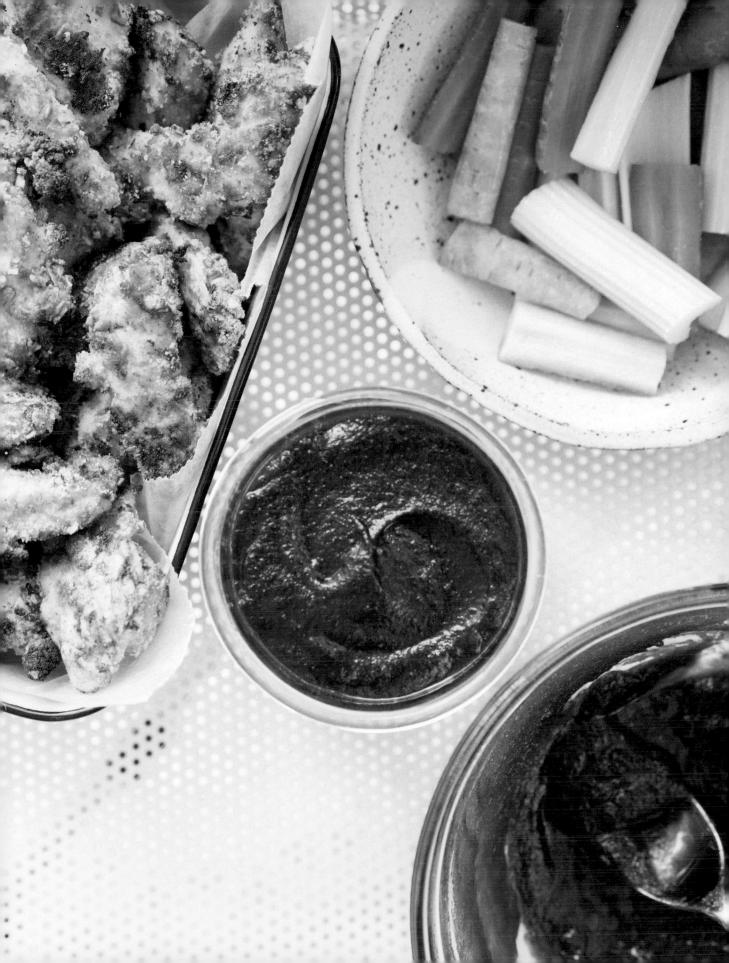

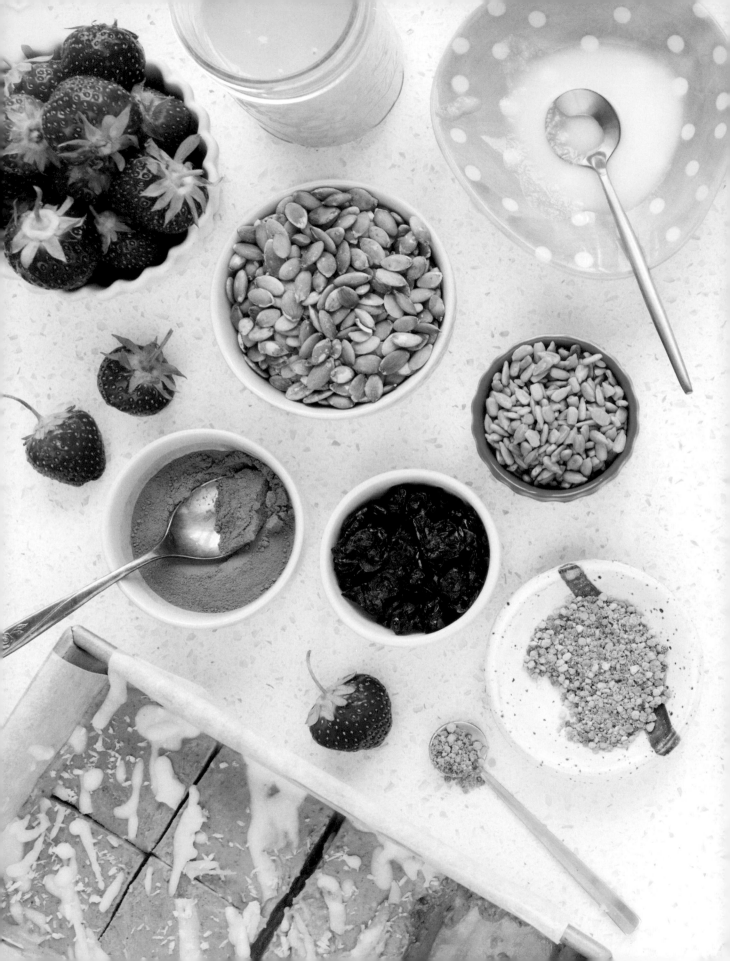

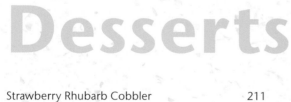

Desserts

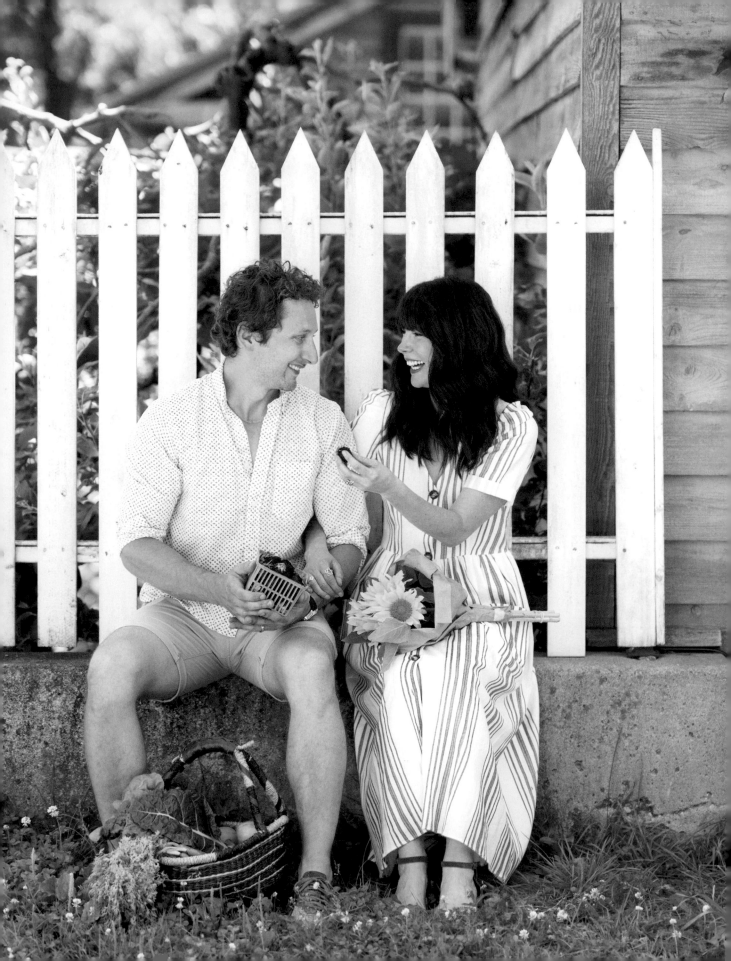

DESSERTS

I've been a dessert lover since a young age. Sunday dinners always included a homemade dessert made by my mom, such as the Peach Coconut Crisp (page 212). We both love to bake and I enjoy eating the results just as much. Dessert is something that should be fully enjoyed, without guilt and without any negative effects. My desserts are absolutely guilt-free and good for you.

In this chapter, you'll soon discover that I love chocolate. People love their daily coffee like I love my daily chocolate fix. In fact, I would totally steal a bite of a Hazelnut Chocolate Tart (page 228) or enjoy a Beet Quinoa Chocolate Cupcake (page 223) slathered with almond butter at breakfast because they are packed with goodness and better than coffee! If you are not a chocolate lover like me, don't worry—you will find lots of non-chocolate treats in this chapter that are still decadent and delicious. Try my Strawberry Rhubarb Cobbler (page 211) or Strawberries and Cream Freezer Fudge (page 239). There is something for everyone!

Don't let the decadence fool you into thinking these desserts are not good for you, because they are packed with whole-food goodness, nut-based flours and natural sweeteners. Whether you are baking just for yourself or for the whole family, I hope you come back to these recipes time and time again, like I do.

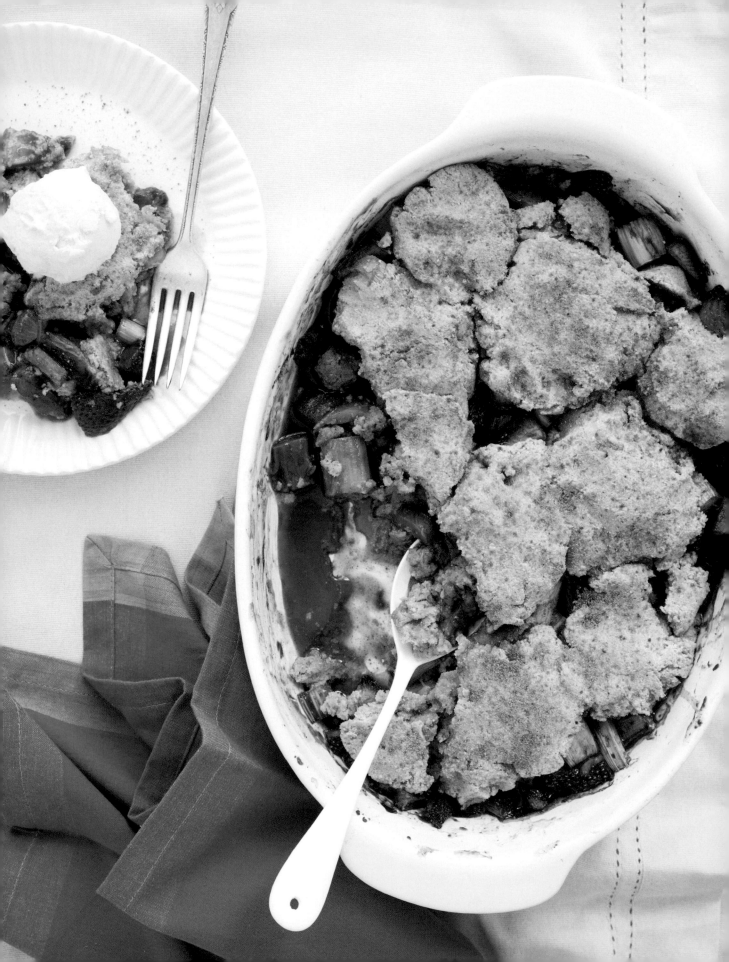

Strawberry Rhubarb Cobbler
Dairy-free • Gluten-free • Grain-free • Kid-friendly • Vegetarian

Serves 6

Every spring I make a dessert with rhubarb, and this cobbler is the ultimate wholesome home-baked dessert you'll want to make over and over again. Rhubarb paired with strawberries is always a winning combination. Both are rich in vitamin C and fibre, so you've got not only a tasty cobbler but a super-healthy one too.

If you're not a fan of rhubarb, you can use any other berry or just increase the strawberries. This cobbler is grain-free and gluten-free, making it ideal for those with food sensitivities. Add a scoop of vanilla coconut milk ice cream and you have the best dessert ever.

Cobbler Topping
1 cup (250 mL) almond flour
   (almond meal)
½ cup (125 mL) coconut flour
1 tablespoon (15 mL) coconut sugar
1 teaspoon (5 mL) baking powder
1 teaspoon (5 mL) cinnamon
4 eggs
½ cup (125 mL) coconut milk
3 tablespoons (45 mL) coconut oil, melted

Strawberry Rhubarb Filling
3 cups (750 mL) chopped fresh or
   thawed frozen strawberries
2 cups (500 mL) chopped fresh or
   thawed frozen rhubarb
¼ cup (60 mL) coconut sugar
1 tablespoon (15 mL) arrowroot
   starch/flour
1 tablespoon (15 mL) cinnamon

1. Preheat the oven to 350°F (180°C). Grease a 13- × 9-inch (3.5 L) baking dish with coconut oil.

2. **Make the Cobbler Topping** In a large bowl, whisk together the almond flour, coconut flour, coconut sugar, baking powder and cinnamon.

3. In a small bowl, whisk together the eggs, coconut milk and coconut oil. Add the wet mixture to the dry mixture and mix until fully combined. The crumble will be slightly dry.

4. **Make the Strawberry Rhubarb Filling** In a large bowl, combine the strawberries and rhubarb. In a small bowl, stir together the coconut sugar, arrowroot starch and cinnamon. Sprinkle this mixture over the strawberry and rhubarb and stir it in. Scrape the filling into the baking dish.

5. Using a large spoon, scoop the cobbler topping evenly over the filling. Using your hands, gently press the topping to flatten it a bit.

6. Bake for 30 to 35 minutes, until the topping is golden brown and a knife inserted in the topping comes out clean. Serve right away or let cool, cover and refrigerate for up to 5 days. Reheat in the oven at 350°F (180°C) for 10 minutes.

Peach Coconut Crisp

Gluten-free • Grain-free • Kid-friendly • Vegetarian

Serves 6

My mom is a total pro when it comes to making a good crisp. Most Sundays she would make a delicious and healthy home-cooked meal complete with a wholesome dessert. Her apple crisp was always amazing! I've taken everything I've learned from my mom and applied it to my own yummy Peach Coconut Crisp.

There is no better time to make a peach crisp than when peaches are in season. However, this crisp works with frozen peaches too. You just have to let the peaches thaw and drain off the juice. No need to peel the peaches if you're using organic. The crisp topping is totally grain-free and gluten-free, and you can make it dairy-free if you use coconut oil instead of butter.

Peach and Coconut Filling

4 cups (1 L) chopped fresh or thawed frozen peaches
2 tablespoons (30 mL) coconut sugar
1 teaspoon (5 mL) cinnamon

Crisp Topping

2½ cups (625 mL) mixed raw pecans, cashews and/or hazelnuts
¼ cup (60 mL) unsweetened shredded coconut
2 tablespoons (30 mL) coconut sugar
1 teaspoon (5 mL) cinnamon
½ teaspoon (2 mL) ground nutmeg
2 tablespoons (30 mL) cold unsalted butter, cubed, or melted coconut oil

1. Preheat the oven to 350°F (180°C). Grease an 8-inch (20 cm) round baking dish with coconut oil.

2. **Make the Peach and Coconut Filling** In a large bowl, stir together the peaches, coconut sugar and cinnamon. Scrape the filling into the baking dish.

3. **Make the Crisp Topping** In a food processor, pulse the nuts until crumbly. Transfer to a medium bowl and add the coconut, coconut sugar, cinnamon, nutmeg and butter.

4. Sprinkle the topping evenly over the filling. Bake for 30 to 35 minutes, until the peaches are fork-tender and the topping is golden. Be careful you don't burn the nuts. Check the crisp after 20 minutes and if the nuts are getting dark, cover the crisp loosely with foil. Serve right away or let cool, then store covered in the fridge for up to 5 days. Reheat in the oven at 350°F (180°C) for 10 minutes.

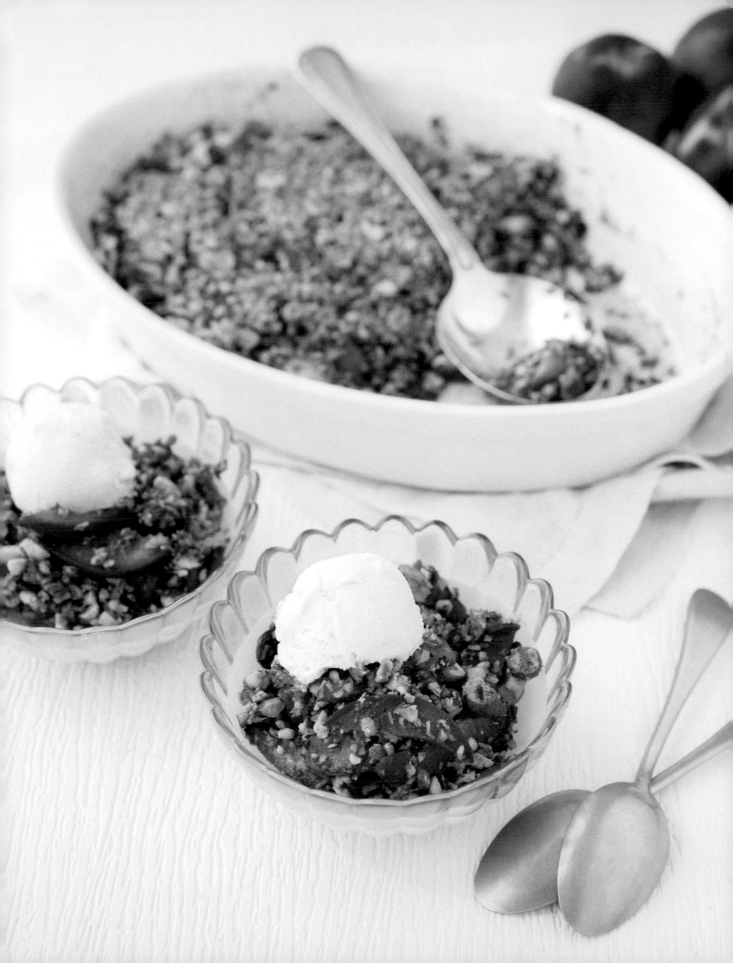

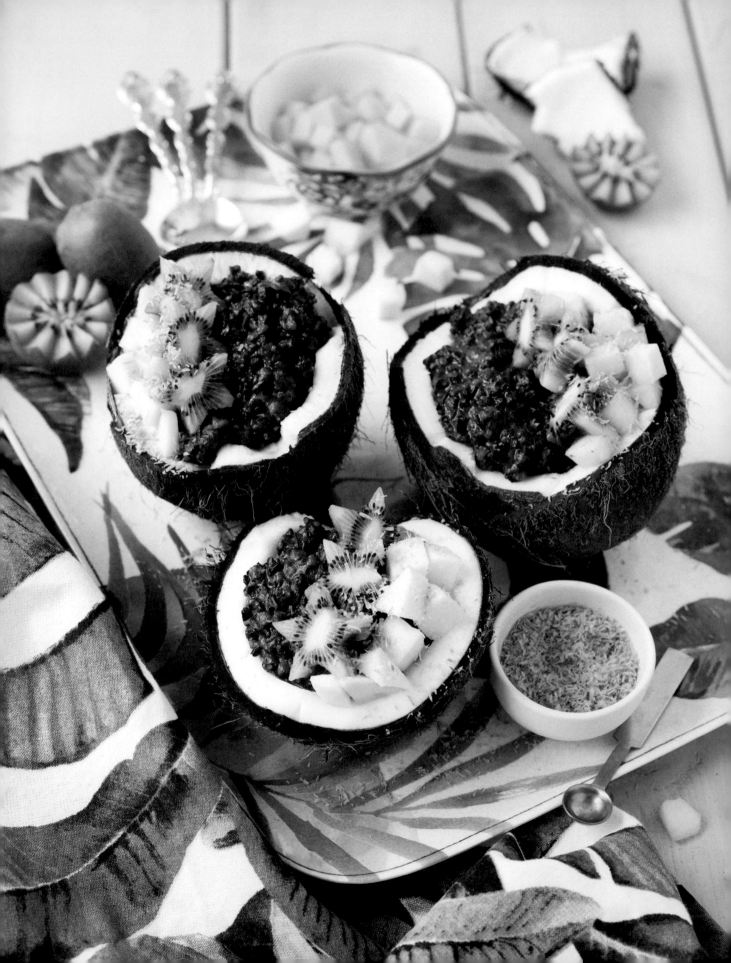

Coconut Black Rice Pudding

Dairy-free · Gluten-free · Kid-friendly · Nut-free · Vegan

Serves 4 to 6

This coconut black rice pudding is creamy, rich and scrumptious, with a distinctive and memorable spiciness from the cardamom. It's a wonderful dessert or a fulfilling breakfast when topped with fresh fruit.

Japonica rice is a combo of black rice and mahogany rice. It has a roasted nutty flavour that lends itself well to the other ingredients. If you can't find it at the health food store, use black rice, which is easy to find in the ethnic section of the grocery store. It's super rich in health-promoting anthocyanins, which are the same antioxidants found in blueberries.

¼ cup (60 mL) unsweetened shredded coconut or coconut flakes
1 cup (250 mL) japonica rice or black rice
2 cups (500 mL) water
1 can (14 ounces/400 mL) full-fat coconut milk
2 tablespoons (30 mL) coconut sugar
½ teaspoon (2 mL) ground cardamom
Diced kiwi and mango, for garnish

1. Preheat the oven to 325°F (160°C). Line a baking sheet with parchment paper.

2. Evenly spread the coconut on the baking sheet. Bake for 5 to 10 minutes, until golden brown.

3. In a medium saucepan, combine the rice and water and bring to a boil. Cover, reduce the heat to low and simmer for 40 minutes. If the rice is still crunchy, add 2 tablespoons (30 mL) water and cook for another 5 to 10 minutes, until the rice fluffs with a fork. Remove from the heat and fluff with a fork.

4. Stir in the coconut milk, coconut sugar and cardamom. Serve warm, garnished with the toasted coconut and fresh fruit.

Blackberry and Strawberry Galette

Gluten-free • Grain-free • Kid-friendly • Vegetarian

Serves 4 to 6

This is the best dessert to win over a crowd of picky eaters who think healthy can't taste good! I used to think galettes were only for pastry chefs, as they looked too complicated to make. But after an entire year of purchasing savoury galettes from my local farmers' market, I decided it was time I learned how to make my own and share it on my blog. It was a hit with my whole family and my blog readers! You'll be happy to know that even if you're not a baker, this recipe is straightforward and foolproof.

Make sure the butter is very cold, which makes the pastry easier to roll out.

Pastry

1½ cups (375 mL) almond flour
   (almond meal)
½ cup (125 mL) tapioca starch/flour
6 tablespoons (90 mL) coconut sugar
1 teaspoon (5 mL) cinnamon
6 tablespoons (90 mL) cold unsalted
   butter, cubed
2 eggs, divided
1 teaspoon (5 mL) coconut sugar (optional)
½ teaspoon (2 mL) cinnamon (optional)

Blackberry and Strawberry Filling

2 cups (500 mL) fresh blackberries,
   cut in half
1 cup (250 mL) chopped fresh strawberries
1 tablespoon (15 mL) lemon zest
1 tablespoon (15 mL) lemon juice

1. **Make the Pastry** In a food processor, combine the almond flour, tapioca starch, coconut sugar, cinnamon and butter. Pulse until the mixture is the texture of coarse meal.

2. Add 1 egg and pulse just until the dough comes together in small chunks. Scrape the dough out onto a work surface and shape into a ball. Flatten into a 5-inch (12 cm) disc, wrap with plastic wrap and chill in the fridge for at least 1 hour or in the freezer for 30 minutes.

3. **Meanwhile, make the Blackberry and Strawberry Filling** In a medium bowl, stir together the blackberries, strawberries, lemon zest and lemon juice. Set aside.

4. Preheat the oven to 375°F (190°C).

5. **Assemble the Galette** On a floured sheet of parchment paper and using a rolling pin sprinkled with flour, roll out the dough into a 10-inch (25 cm) circle. It's okay if it's not perfectly shaped. Slide the pastry, on the parchment paper, onto a baking sheet.

6. Spread the fruit filling in the centre of the dough, stopping 2 to 2½ inches (5 to 6 cm) from the edge. Fold the dough border up over the sides, overlapping in pleats here and there. Don't worry if the dough cracks as you fold it. Just press the dough with your fingers to seal the crack. It doesn't have to look perfect.

7. In a small bowl, whisk the remaining egg. Brush the folded-over dough with the egg wash for a golden top edge. Sprinkle the pastry border with coconut sugar and cinnamon, if using. Bake for 35 minutes, or until the crust is golden brown. Enjoy immediately or store covered in the fridge for up to 5 days.

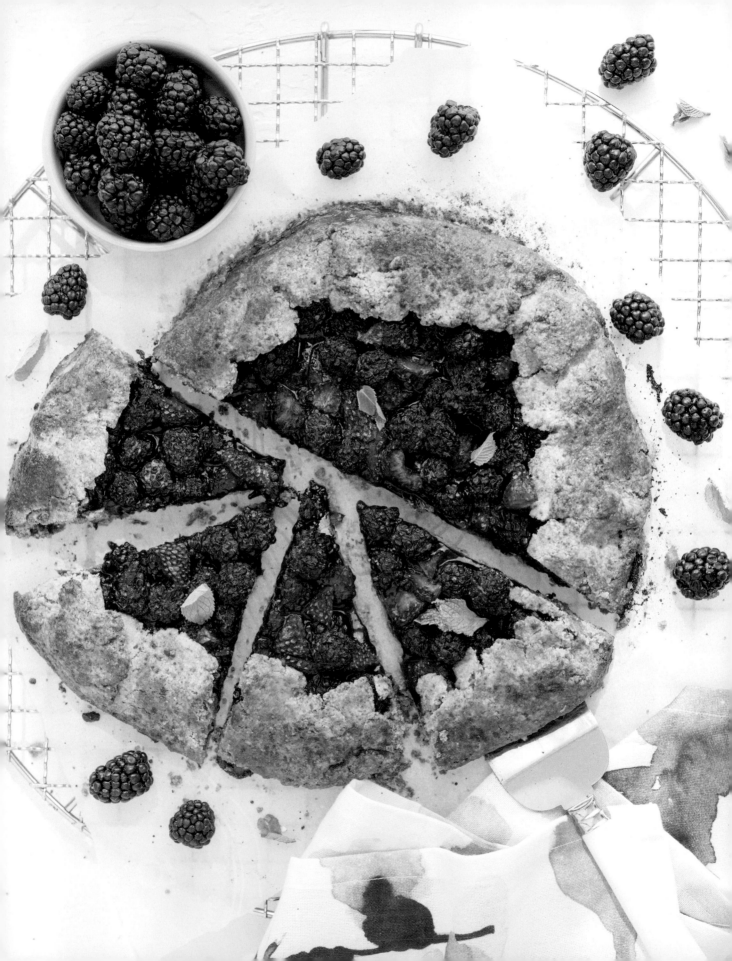

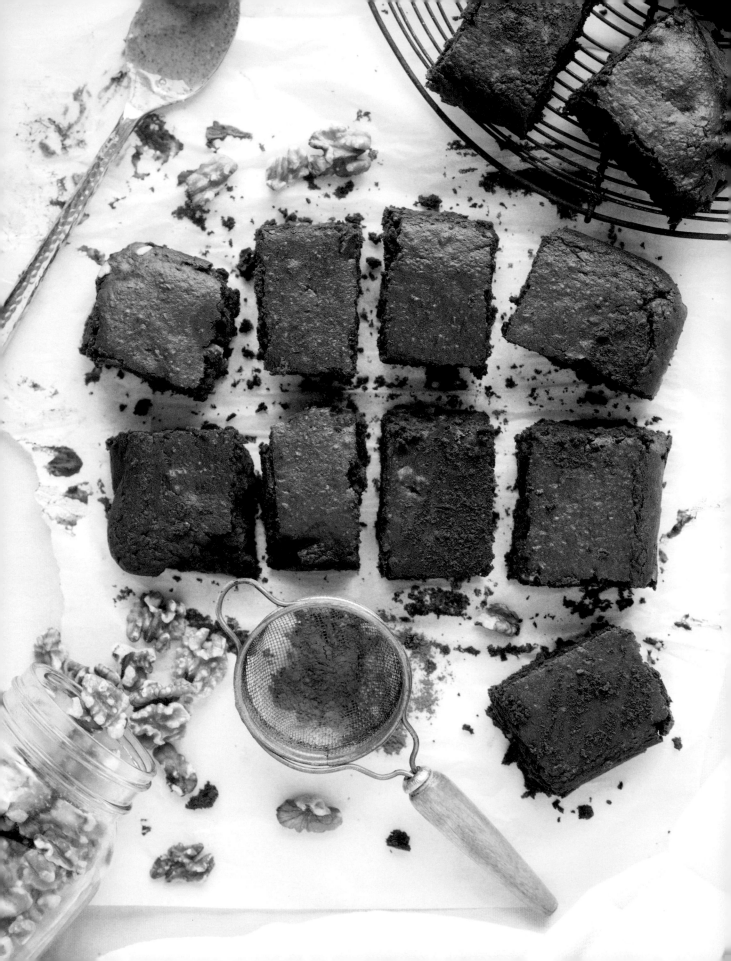

Chickpea Walnut Brownies

Dairy-free • Gluten-free • Grain-free • Kid-friendly • Vegetarian

Makes 12 brownies

These brownies are everything you want a brownie to be: fudgy, sweet (but not over-the-top sweet), with a little crunch from the walnuts. The best part is that you'll be feeling great after eating them because there is no refined sugar to send your blood sugar on a rollercoaster. They are packed with tons of fibre, plant-based protein, iron, magnesium, and calcium and they support digestive health.

The star ingredient in these brownies is the chickpeas. Research has shown that when people consume chickpeas they feel more "satisfied" overall. This means if you have one of these brownies as a power snack, you're more likely to feel satiated, especially if you slather it with some almond butter. If you're packing a nut-free lunchbox, simply omit the walnuts.

4 Medjool dates, pitted
1 can (14 ounces/398 mL) chickpeas, drained and rinsed
½ cup (125 mL) real maple syrup
⅓ cup (75 mL) coconut oil, melted
1 egg
1 teaspoon (5 mL) pure vanilla extract
½ cup (125 mL) raw cacao powder
1 teaspoon (5 mL) baking powder
½ teaspoon (2 mL) fine sea salt
½ cup (125 mL) chopped raw walnuts
½ cup (125 mL) semi-sweet dairy-free chocolate chips

1. Preheat the oven to 350°F (180°C). Line the bottom and sides of an 8-inch (2 L) square baking pan with parchment paper or grease with coconut oil.

2. Soak the dates in hot water for 10 minutes, then drain.

3. In a food processor, combine the dates, chickpeas, maple syrup, coconut oil, egg and vanilla. Pulse until fully combined.

4. In a small bowl, stir together the cacao powder, baking powder and sea salt. Add to the chickpea mixture and pulse to combine.

5. Remove the blade from the food processor and fold in the walnuts and chocolate chips. Scrape the batter into the prepared pan. Bake for 20 minutes, or until a fork inserted in the centre of the brownies comes out clean.

6. Let cool in the pan on a rack for 10 minutes. Remove from the pan to cool completely before cutting into 12 squares. Store, wrapped well with plastic wrap, in the fridge for up to 1 week or in the freezer for up to 3 months.

Almond Butter Rice Crispy Squares

Dairy-free · Gluten-free · Kid-friendly · Vegetarian

Makes 9 squares

Throughout my teens and my twenties, I used to make rice crispy squares the old-fashioned way a few times every month. I will admit they didn't make me feel great, and it was impossible to eat only one square because the refined sugar turned me into a sugar-eating monster! Fast-forward to today and I've got the next best thing: a healthy alternative to a favourite treat.

These squares are packed with wholesome goodness—although they are still pretty addictive. The almond butter makes them very satisfying and much more filling. It's important to use a super-sticky natural sweetener like brown rice syrup or coconut nectar so that the squares stay together. Both can be found in the natural foods section of your grocery store or the health food store. If you plan on serving these at a picnic or barbecue—which I highly recommend, especially if there are kids around—they are best served chilled, otherwise they are a sticky mess!

½ cup (125 mL) brown rice syrup or
   coconut nectar
½ cup (125 mL) natural almond butter
2 tablespoons (30 mL) coconut oil (solid)
3½ cups (875 mL) brown rice crisp cereal
½ cup (125 mL) dairy-free mini chocolate
   chips, divided

1. Line the bottom and sides of an 8-inch (2 L) square baking pan with parchment paper.

2. In a medium saucepan, combine the brown rice syrup, almond butter and coconut oil. Stir over low heat until the coconut oil is melted and the mixture is combined. Remove from the heat and let cool slightly so the chocolate chips don't melt when you mix everything together.

3. Pour the rice crisp cereal into a large bowl. Pour the rice syrup mixture over the cereal and stir until well combined. Fold in ¼ cup (60 mL) of the chocolate chips. Scrape the mixture into the prepared pan and evenly spread it with a spatula.

4. In a small pot, stir the remaining ¼ cup (60 mL) chocolate chips over low heat until melted. Drizzle the melted chocolate over the rice crispy squares. Cover with plastic wrap and refrigerate for at least 2 hours.

5. When ready to serve, cut into 9 squares. Store in an airtight container in the fridge for up to 1 week.

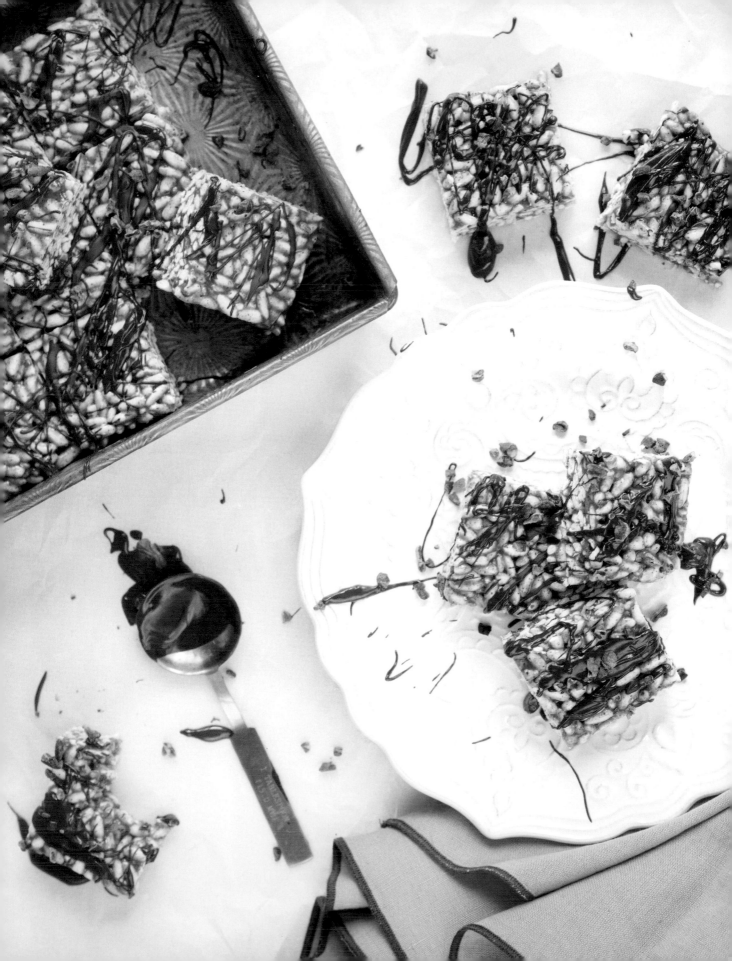

Beet Quinoa Chocolate Cupcakes

Dairy-free • Gluten-free • Kid-friendly • Nut-free • Vegetarian

Makes 18 mini cupcakes

This recipe originated from Ma McCarthy's Chocolate Quinoa Cake, which has been hugely popular on my blog for several years and is made for pretty much every birthday in our home. You'd never know something as healthy as beets were an ingredient in these cupcakes! I turned the original cake recipe into cupcakes because they're easier for little people and, well, this way I have an excuse to eat more than one! I have never added icing because I find these are sweet enough on their own, but you could melt some coconut butter and spread it on top of the cupcakes. They are also delicious with a dollop of almond butter.

Cooking the beets ahead of time will make the prep much faster. I peel the beets (only for this recipe), cut them into chunks, place them on a baking sheet lined with parchment paper and roast them at 350°F (180°C) for about 45 minutes or until fork-tender.

⅔ cup (150 mL) white quinoa
1⅓ cups (325 mL) water
1 cup (250 mL) peeled cooked red
   beets, cut into chunks
4 eggs
½ cup (125 mL) coconut oil, melted
¼ cup (60 mL) real maple syrup
1 cup (250 mL) raw cacao powder
   or unsweetened cocoa powder
½ cup (125 mL) coconut sugar
1 teaspoon (5 mL) baking powder
1 teaspoon (5 mL) baking soda
⅓ cup (75 mL) dairy-free mini
   chocolate chips

1. Preheat the oven to 350°F (180°C). Line a mini muffin tin with paper liners.

2. In a medium saucepan, combine the quinoa and water and bring to a boil. Reduce the heat and simmer, with the lid slightly ajar, for 15 minutes, or until the quinoa is fluffy. Remove from the heat.

3. In a food processor, combine the cooked quinoa, beets, eggs, coconut oil, maple syrup, cacao powder, coconut sugar, baking powder and baking soda. Pulse until smooth. Remove the blade and fold in the mini chocolate chips.

4. Divide the batter among the muffin cups. Bake for 18 minutes, or until the tops have a few cracks and a fork inserted in the centre of a cupcake comes out clean.

5. Let cool in the tin for 5 minutes. Tip out the cupcakes and transfer to a rack to cool completely. Store in an airtight container in the fridge for up to 1 week or in a resealable plastic freezer bag in the freezer for up to 3 months.

Dark Chocolate Superfood Bars

Dairy-free • Gluten-free • Grain-free • Kid-friendly • Vegetarian

Makes 6 to 8 bars

If you're a chocolate lover like me, you will love these bars—truly addictive! They are the ultimate chocolate lover's treat because they are so rich and satisfying with a perfect combination of crunch, chew and melt-in-your-mouth goodness. Pure bliss!

You can use roasted cocoa powder in place of raw cacao, but I highly recommend raw cacao. It is one of nature's most beloved superfoods. It is rich in flavanols, a group of antioxidant phytochemicals that protect heart health. The less refined the cacao, the more flavonoids present, which is why raw is best. Raw cacao is also rich in magnesium, a mineral essential for a healthy nervous system. My only caution is that raw cacao powder can be stimulating for children. You know your child best, but if you have a child that's sensitive to chocolate, they may be up all night if they eat a whole bar.

½ cup + 3 tablespoons (170 mL) coconut oil

1 cup (250 mL) raw cacao powder

⅓ cup (75 mL) real maple syrup

2 tablespoons (30 mL) of your favourite unsweetened nut milk

½ teaspoon (2 mL) cinnamon

1 tablespoon (15 mL) chia seeds

2 tablespoons (30 mL) raw pumpkin seeds, divided

2 tablespoons (30 mL) raw sunflower seeds, divided

2 tablespoons (30 mL) hemp seeds, divided

2 tablespoons (30 mL) dried cranberries, divided

1 tablespoon (15 mL) bee pollen

1. In a medium saucepan, melt the coconut oil over low heat. Stir in the cacao powder and maple syrup. Once fully combined, add the nut milk and cinnamon and stir. Be careful not to burn the mixture.

2. Add the chia seeds and 1 tablespoon (15 mL) each of the pumpkins seeds, sunflower seeds, hemp seeds and cranberries. Stir well.

3. Line a 8½- × 4½-inch (1.5 L) loaf pan with parchment paper, leaving extra paper to overhang to make it easier to remove the bars once set.

4. Pour the mixture into the pan and smooth the top, if necessary. Sprinkle with the remaining 1 tablespoon (15 mL) each of the pumpkin seeds, sunflower seeds, hemp seeds and cranberries, then sprinkle with bee pollen. Cover with plastic wrap and freeze for 4 hours or overnight.

5. To serve, remove from the freezer and let sit for 5 minutes before slicing. Using the overhanging parchment paper, lift the bars out of the pan. Slice into 1-inch (2.5 cm) bars or 2-inch (5 cm) squares. Store wrapped individually and freeze in a resealable plastic freezer bag for up to 3 months.

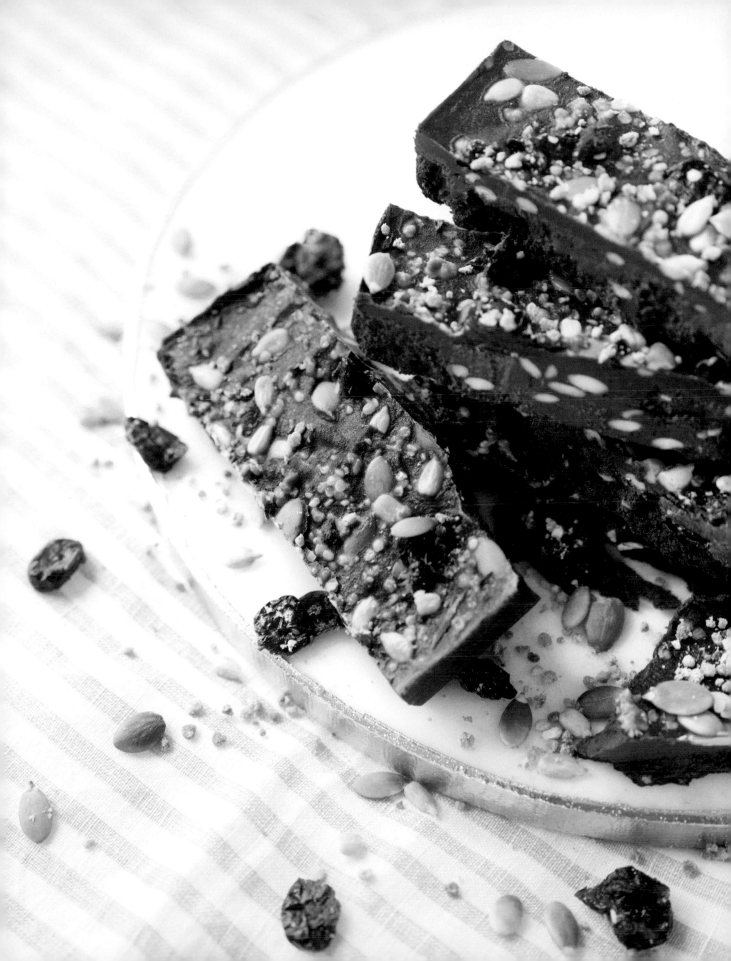

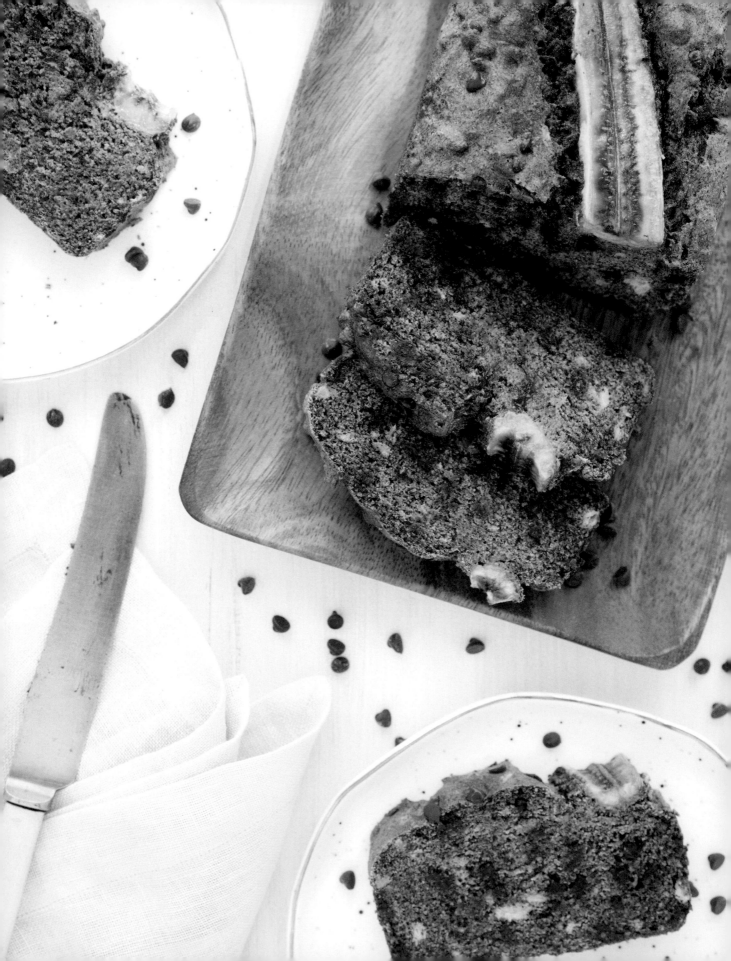

Buckwheat Chocolate Chip Banana Bread

Dairy-free • Gluten-free • Kid-friendly • Vegetarian

Makes 1 loaf

If you have a bunch of ripe bananas sitting on your kitchen counter, then you've got a reason to make this banana bread! Bananas are always on my grocery list because of the number of smoothies I make in a week, but I always check the discount rack at the grocery store for ripe bananas because they are often 50 percent off. That gives me the perfect excuse to make banana bread (as if I need an excuse!).

The main ingredient aside from bananas is buckwheat flour. Despite its name, this flour is gluten-free and it adds an earthy flavour to this bread. Light-coloured buckwheat flour is my preference because its flavour is more mild, but sometimes the package isn't labelled "light" or "dark." The maple syrup is optional. Often I don't add it because the bananas are sweet enough on their own, but it's up to you.

1 cup (250 mL) buckwheat flour
1 teaspoon (5 mL) baking soda
½ teaspoon (2 mL) baking powder
¼ teaspoon (1 mL) sea salt
2 eggs
3 ripe bananas, mashed
3 tablespoons (45 mL) of your favourite unsweetened nut milk
3 tablespoons (45 mL) real maple syrup (optional)
2 tablespoons + 1½ teaspoons (37 mL) coconut oil, melted
1 teaspoon (5 mL) pure vanilla extract
½ cup (125 mL) dairy-free mini chocolate chips

1. Preheat the oven to 350°F (180°C). Grease an 8½- × 4½-inch (1.5 L) loaf pan with coconut oil.

2. In a large bowl, whisk together the buckwheat flour, baking soda, baking powder and sea salt.

3. In a medium bowl, whisk the eggs, then whisk in the bananas, nut milk, maple syrup (if using), coconut oil and vanilla. Add the wet mixture to the dry mixture and stir until combined. Fold in the chocolate chips.

4. Scrape the batter into the prepared loaf pan. Bake for 30 to 35 minutes, until a knife inserted in the centre of the loaf comes out clean.

5. Let cool in the pan on a rack for 10 minutes. Turn the loaf out of the pan onto a rack to cool completely before slicing. Store in an airtight container in the fridge for up to 1 week or slice, wrap individually and freeze in a resealable plastic freezer bag for up to 3 months.

Hazelnut Chocolate Tarts

Dairy-free • Gluten-free • Grain-free • Kid-friendly • Vegan

Makes six 3- to 4-inch (8 to 10 cm) tarts

My passion for chocolate met with hazelnuts and fireworks happened! I know this combination is as old as it gets, but for me the deliciousness and the enjoyment of it never gets old. Creamy and rich, with the perfect level of sweetness, these hazelnut chocolate tarts are everything! This no-bake, no-fuss recipe is a secret weapon if you're wanting to impress someone. They will think you slaved for hours, yet no one will know how easy these tarts are, and healthy to boot! Your secret is safe with me. These are quite filling from the hazelnut butter, coconut milk and nutty crust, so they're perfect for sharing if you're so inclined.

Make sure to use full-fat coconut milk for the best result. You'll love that you don't need to soak the cashews, because there is enough liquid from the coconut milk—time saver! If you don't have individual tart pans, you can make this in an 8-inch (20 cm) springform pan. Some children are sensitive to raw cacao and it can be stimulating for them. Keep this in mind if you plan on serving this to a young child.

Crunchy Chocolate Crust

2 cups (500 mL) raw pecans
½ cup (125 mL) unsweetened coconut flakes
¼ cup (60 mL) raw cacao nibs
2 tablespoons (30 mL) coconut oil, melted
15 to 20 soft Medjool dates, pitted

Hazelnut Chocolate Filling

2 cups (500 mL) raw cashews
½ cup (125 mL) raw cacao powder
½ cup (125 mL) real maple syrup
¼ cup (60 mL) natural hazelnut butter
1 can (14 ounces/400 mL) full-fat coconut milk
½ cup (125 mL) chopped raw hazelnuts, for garnish

1. **Make the Crunchy Chocolate Crust** In a food processor, combine the pecans, coconut flakes, cacao nibs, coconut oil and 15 dates. Pulse until crumbly. The mixture should be sticky. If not, you can add more dates and pulse again. (You want the crust mixture to stick together when pressed into the tart pan.)

2. Evenly divide the nut mixture among six 3- to 4-inch (8 to 10 cm) tart pans. Press it in firmly, making sure the sides are well packed and the base is relatively even. Refrigerate while you make the filling.

3. **Make the Hazelnut Chocolate Filling** In a high-speed blender, combine the cashews, cacao powder, maple syrup, hazelnut butter and coconut milk. Blend until smooth. Divide the filling among the tart shells. Freeze for 4 to 6 hours.

4. To serve, remove the tarts from the freezer and let sit for 15 minutes, then pop the tarts out of the pans. Sprinkle with chopped hazelnuts just before serving. Store, tightly wrapped in plastic wrap, in a resealable plastic freezer bag in the freezer for up to 3 months.

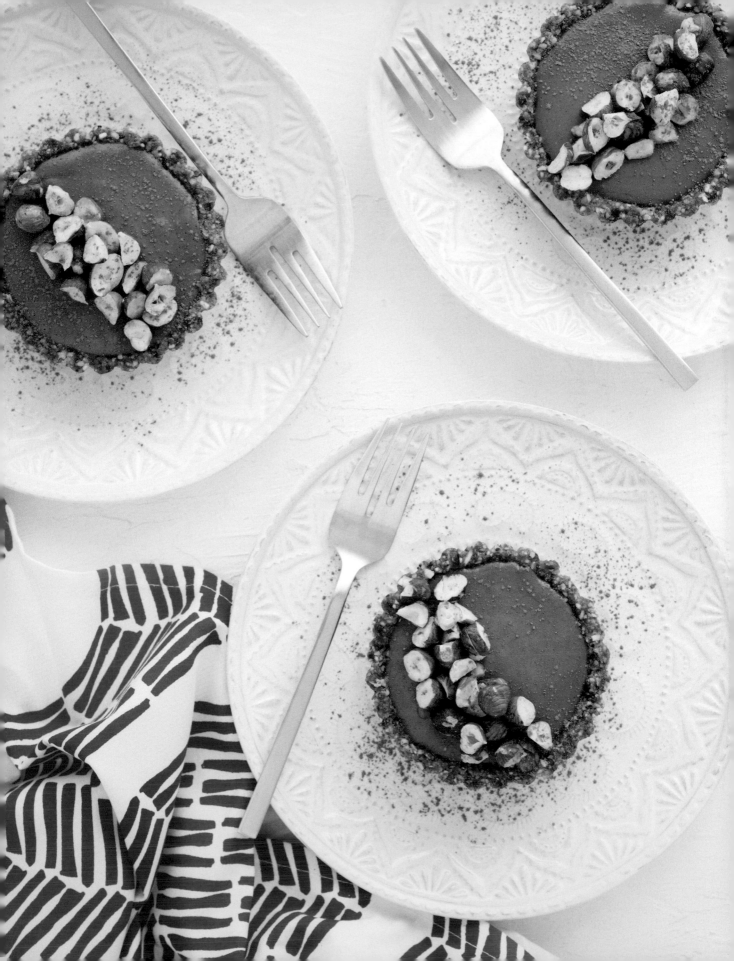

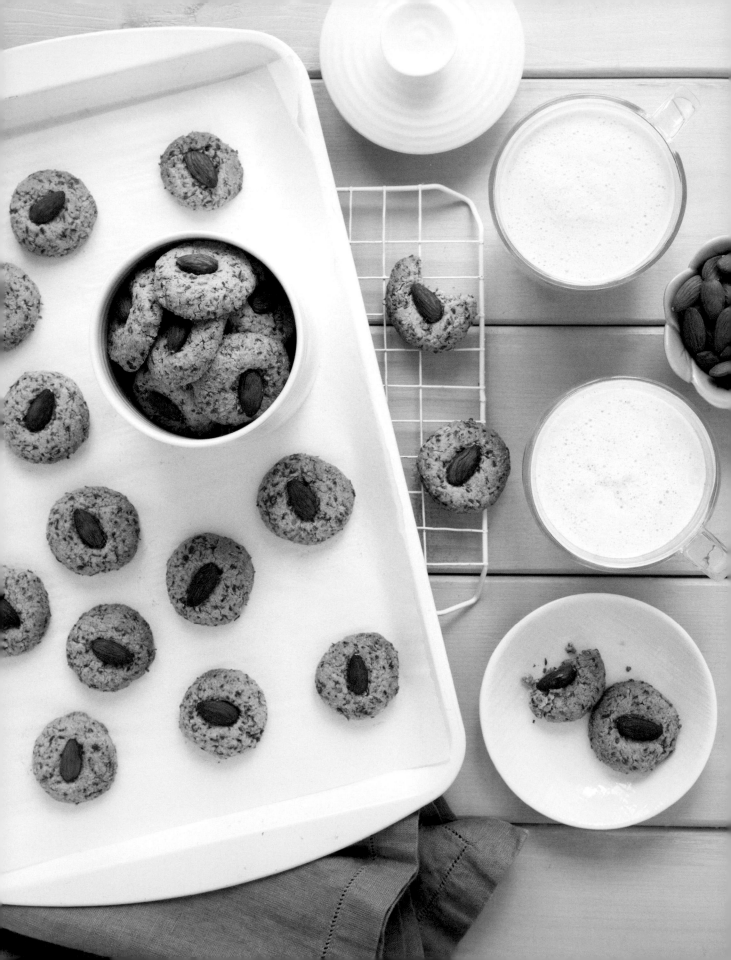

Joyous Amaretti

Dairy-free • Gluten-free • Grain-free • Kid-friendly • Vegan

Makes 24 cookies

Amaretti are a classic Italian cookie that I absolutely love, but unfortunately they are full of white sugar. Of course my version contains no white sugar whatsoever! Plus they are paleo and vegan. As much as I like to practise mindfulness when eating, it's hard not to eat several of these cookies in one sitting!

I first made these cookies totally by accident. I didn't have all the ingredients to make another cookie recipe, but while rummaging through my fridge I discovered I had some almond extract, which really enhances the almond flavour, and flaxseeds to boost the fibre. To my surprise, I was thrilled by the first one I tasted, because they reminded me so much of amaretti but were a healthy joyous version. Now, I don't want to mess with your Nonna's recipe, but I encourage you to make these for her and then let me know what she says!

1½ cups (375 mL) almond flour
   (almond meal)
½ cup (125 mL) ground flaxseed
   (flax meal)
½ cup (125 mL) coconut oil, melted
¼ cup (60 mL) natural almond butter
¼ cup (60 mL) real maple syrup
1 teaspoon (5 mL) pure almond extract
24 whole raw almonds

1. Preheat the oven to 350°F (180°C). Line a baking sheet with parchment paper or grease with coconut oil.

2. In a medium bowl, combine the almond flour, flaxseed, coconut oil, almond butter, maple syrup and almond extract. Stir until well mixed.

3. Using about 1 heaping tablespoon (18 mL) of the mixture at a time, roll between your hands into 1-inch (2.5 cm) balls. Place them about 1 inch (2.5 cm) apart on the prepared baking sheet. Flatten the dough balls with your hand so that they are about ½ inch (1 cm) thick and place an almond on top of each cookie.

4. Bake for 8 for 10 minutes, until the cookies are golden brown on the outside and soft in the centre. Do not overcook—you want them soft and chewy on the inside.

5. Let cool on the baking sheet for 2 minutes. Transfer the cookies to a rack and cool for at least 10 minutes before serving. Store in an airtight container in the fridge for up to 1 week or in a resealable plastic freezer bag in the freezer for up to 3 months.

Chocolate Chip Oatmeal Tahini Cookies

Dairy-free • Kid-friendly • Nut-free • Vegan

Makes 24 cookies

These cookies have been a blog reader favourite for many years. I think one reason people love these cookies so much—aside from how yummy they are—is because it's a really easy recipe. This recipe is on regular rotation in our home.

Tahini can vary greatly in texture, from thin and creamy to thick and on the dry side, but you can always add a bit more tahini if the batter seems dry. You don't need to shape these into perfect balls either. Just as long as you get a spoonful on the baking sheet, you have cookies!

2 cups (500 mL) old-fashioned rolled oats
   or oat flakes
⅔ cup (150 mL) tahini
⅔ cup (150 mL) dairy-free mini chocolate
   chips
½ cup (125 mL) real maple syrup
1 tablespoon (15 mL) cinnamon
¼ teaspoon (1 mL) sea salt

1. Preheat the oven to 350°F (180°C). Line a baking sheet with parchment paper.

2. In a large bowl, combine the oats, tahini, chocolate chips, maple syrup, cinnamon and sea salt. Stir until fully combined. Make sure the tahini is evenly spread throughout the dough.

3. Scoop 1 heaping tablespoon (18 mL) of dough for each cookie and drop onto the baking sheet, leaving 1 inch (2.5 cm) between the cookies. Bake for 10 to 12 minutes, until the edges are golden brown.

4. Let the cookies cool slightly on the baking sheet, then transfer them to a rack to cool completely. Store in an airtight container in the fridge for up to 1 week or in a resealable plastic freezer bag in the freezer for up to 3 months.

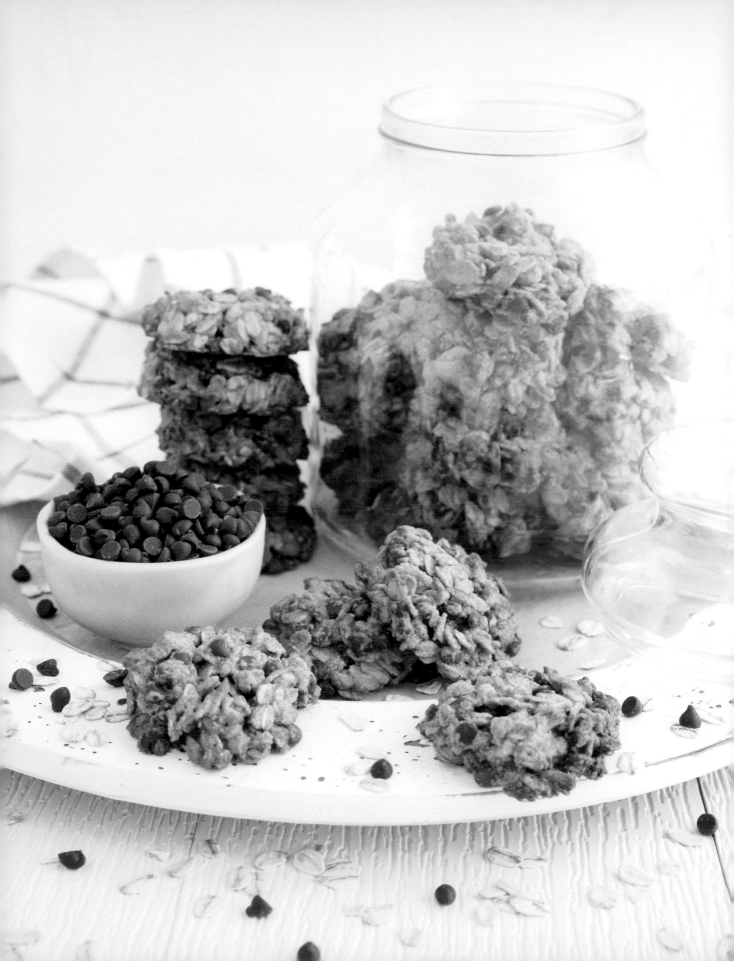

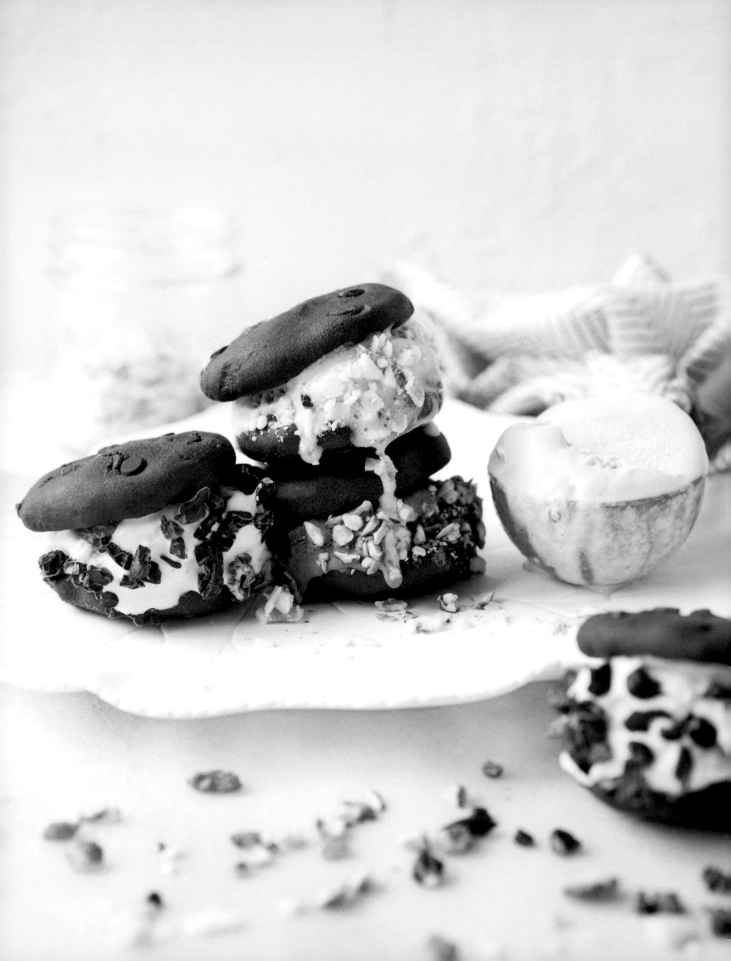

Double Chocolate Chip Ice Cream Sammies

Dairy-free • Gluten-free • Kid-friendly • Vegetarian

Makes 20 cookies, for 10 ice cream sandwiches

These ice cream sandwiches are the ultimate summer treat! What these cookies lack in sweetness is made up for by the ice cream you spread between them. If you plan on making the cookies without turning them into ice cream sandwiches, then you may want to add more maple syrup to the batter.

Brown rice flour yields a denser cookie than average, but they are the perfect sturdiness to hold the sandwich together. These melt fast, so be ready to enjoy them as soon as they are made. You can also make them ahead and store in the freezer tightly wrapped. Remove from the freezer just before serving them.

Dark Chocolate Chip Cookies

1¾ cups (425 mL) brown rice flour
⅔ cup (150 mL) raw cacao powder
1 teaspoon (5 mL) baking powder
2 eggs
½ cup (125 mL) real maple syrup
¼ cup (60 mL) coconut oil, melted
1 teaspoon (5 mL) pure vanilla extract
⅓ cup (75 mL) dairy-free mini chocolate
   chips

Ice Cream Filling and Extras

¼ cup (60 mL) chopped raw pistachios
¼ cup (60 mL) dairy-free mini chocolate
   chips or unsweetened shredded coconut
1 pint (500 mL) of your favourite coconut
   milk ice cream

1. **Make the Dark Chocolate Chip Cookies** Preheat the oven to 350°F (180°C). Line a baking sheet with parchment paper or grease with coconut oil.

2. In a medium bowl, whisk together the brown rice flour, cacao powder and baking powder.

3. In a small bowl, whisk together the eggs, maple syrup, coconut oil and vanilla. Add the wet mixture to the dry mixture and stir to combine. Fold in the chocolate chips.

4. Using 1 heaping tablespoon (18 mL) of the mixture at a time, roll between your hands into 1½-inch (4 cm) balls. Place them about 1 inch (2.5 cm) apart on the prepared baking sheet. You should have 20 balls. If the mixture starts to stick, cool your hands with a little water. Flatten the dough balls with your hand so that they are about ½ inch (1 cm) thick.

5. Bake for 10 to 12 minutes, until they crack a bit on top. The raw cacao makes these dark brown in colour, so you can't judge doneness by colour. Transfer the cookies to a rack to cool completely.

6. **Assemble the Ice Cream Sammies** In a shallow bowl, combine the pistachios and chocolate chips. Using an ice-cream scoop or spoon, scoop 2 to 3 tablespoons (30 to 45 mL) of ice cream and evenly distribute over the flat side of one cookie; top with a second cookie, flat side down. If necessary, squeeze gently so the ice cream spreads to the edges. Roll the sides of the cookies in the pistachio mixture and enjoy immediately before they melt or freeze until ready to serve. Freeze any extra ice cream sandwiches on a baking sheet, then transfer to a resealable plastic freezer bag and freeze for up to 1 month.

Matcha Ice Cream Cake
Dairy-free • Gluten-free • Grain-free • Kid-friendly • Vegetarian

Makes one 8-inch (20 cm) round cake, serves 6 to 8

My love affair with matcha (green tea powder) started decades ago with green tea ice cream at Japanese restaurants. After that I moved on to matcha lattes made with coconut milk, and then I decided it was time to take my loves of ice cream and matcha and combine them. This cake was a total experiment but it was absolute heaven the first time I made it. Since then, I've made it countless times. In fact, it's a wonderful birthday cake!

I typically use 3 tablespoons (45 mL) of high-quality matcha, but if you're a newbie try it first with 2 tablespoons (30 mL), give it a taste and decide if you want to add more. I highly recommend full-fat coconut milk from a can. If you don't use full-fat, the ice cream cake has more of an icy texture than creamy. And creamy is what you want for an ice cream cake!

Chocolate Crust
2 cups (500 mL) raw pecans and/or almonds
½ cup (125 mL) unsweetened shredded coconut
½ cup (125 mL) raw cacao nibs
1 teaspoon (5 mL) cinnamon
12 soft Medjool dates, pitted
1 to 2 tablespoons (15 to 30 mL) water, only as needed if dough is too dry

Matcha Filling
1 cup (250 mL) raw cashews, soaked for at least 4 hours, drained and rinsed
1 cup (250 mL) unsweetened coconut flakes
2 cans (14 ounces/400 mL each) full-fat coconut milk
½ cup (125 mL) pure liquid honey or real maple syrup
2 to 3 tablespoons (30 to 45 mL) matcha (green tea powder)
Fresh berries, for garnish

1. **Make the Chocolate Crust** In a food processor, combine the pecans, coconut, cacao nibs, cinnamon and dates. Pulse until combined and crumbly. (If the mixture is too dry, add the water 1 tablespoon at a time, as needed.)

2. Scrape the mixture into an 8-inch (2 L) springform pan and press it in firmly with your hands, making sure the sides are well packed, about ½ inch (1 cm) up the sides of the pan, and the base is relatively even throughout. Store in the fridge while you make the filling.

3. **Make the Matcha Filling** In a high-speed blender, combine the cashews, coconut flakes, coconut milk, honey and matcha. Blend until very smooth. Pour the filling into the crust. Cover with plastic wrap and freeze for at least 6 hours or overnight.

4. To serve, remove from the freezer and let stand for 15 or 20 minutes before removing the sides of the pan and slicing the cake. Serve topped with fresh berries. Store leftovers, wrapped in plastic wrap, in the freezer for up to 3 months.

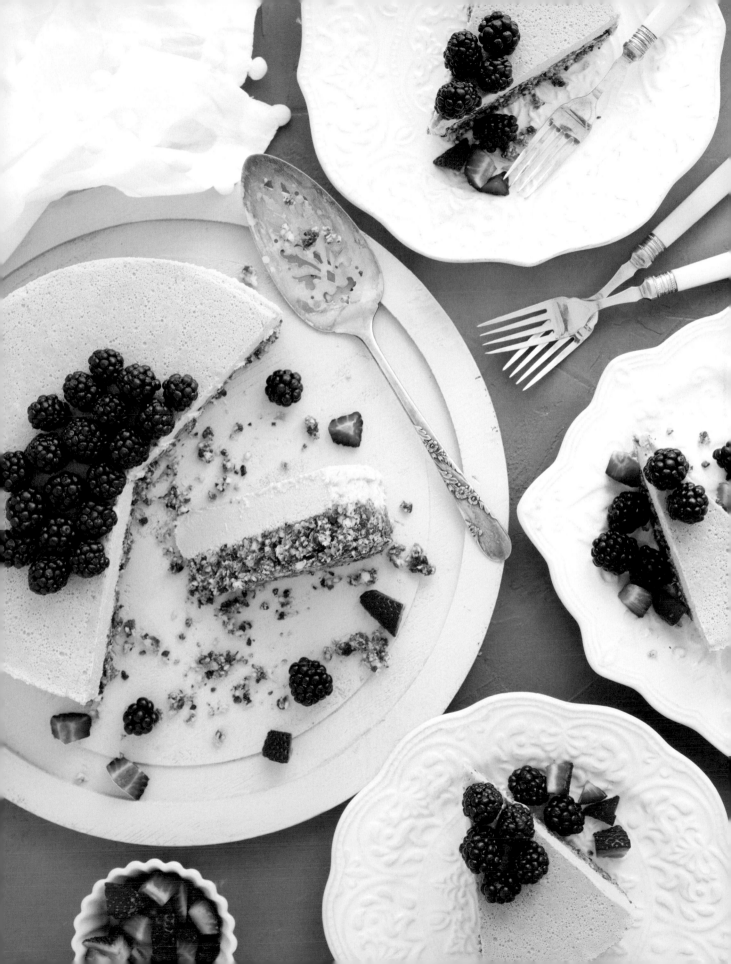

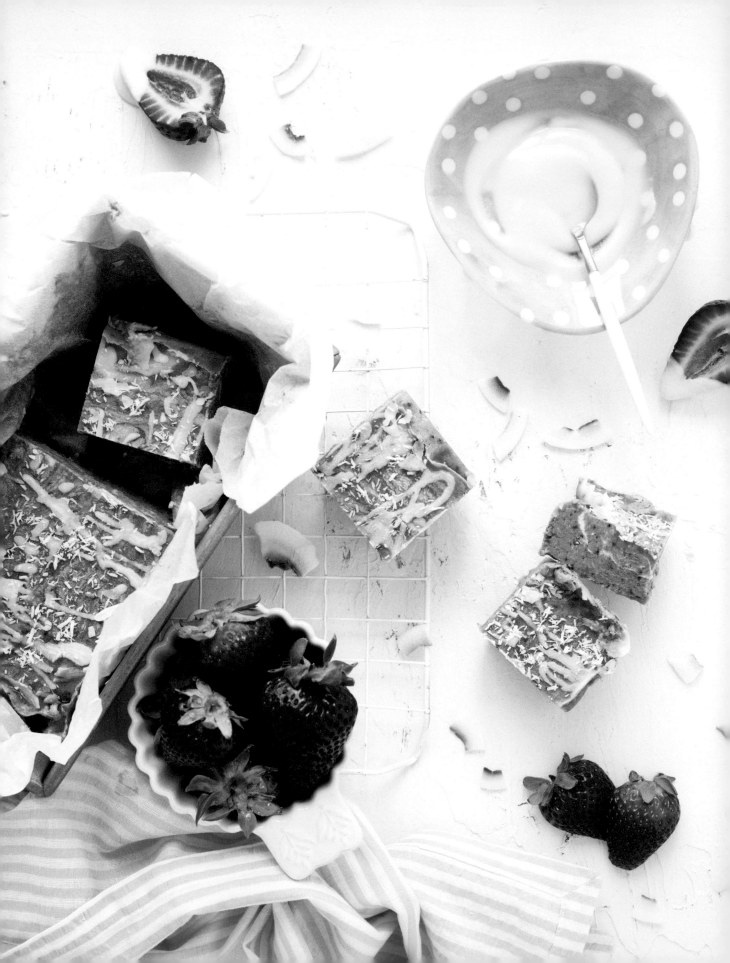

Strawberries and Cream Freezer Fudge

Dairy-free · Gluten-free · Grain-free · Kid-friendly · Nut-free · Vegan

Makes 8 squares

This no-bake, no-fuss dessert is dairy-free, yet it's creamy and oh so good! If you've never used tahini in something sweet before, you're in for a real treat. It has a mild nutty flavour, and it's creamy and rich. Naturally sweetened with maple syrup, this is a healthy dessert staple for summer barbecues—assuming you have a freezer nearby, because this needs to be kept in the freezer until about 15 minutes before serving.

Coconut butter can be found in the natural foods section of your grocery store or the health food store. It's different from coconut oil, in that it's made from ground coconut flesh and includes the fibre and fat.

⅓ cup (75 mL) coconut oil
4 tablespoons (60 mL) coconut butter, divided
3 cups (750 mL) fresh or thawed frozen strawberries
½ cup (125 mL) tahini
¼ cup (60 mL) real maple syrup
1 teaspoon (5 mL) pure vanilla extract
2 tablespoons (30 mL) unsweetened coconut flakes

1. Line the bottom and sides of an 8½- × 4½-inch (1.5 L) loaf pan with parchment paper.

2. In a small pot, combine the coconut oil and 3 tablespoons (45 mL) of the coconut butter. Heat over low heat until the coconut butter just softens. Be careful not to burn the coconut butter.

3. Transfer the coconut mixture to a high-speed blender or food processor. Add the strawberries, tahini, maple syrup and vanilla. Pulse until smooth. Scrape the mixture into the prepared loaf pan.

4. In the same saucepan, melt the remaining 1 tablespoon (15 mL) coconut butter over low heat. Drizzle the melted coconut butter over the berry mixture. Evenly sprinkle the coconut flakes on top. Cover with plastic wrap and freeze for at least 5 hours or overnight.

5. Remove from the freezer 15 minutes before cutting into squares and serving. Store in a resealable plastic freezer bag in the freezer for up to 3 months.

ACKNOWLEDGMENTS

This first person I would like to acknowledge is you. Whether you're familiar with my blog, *Joyous Health*, and my previous books or you're brand new to the joyous healthy way of eating, thank you for picking up this book and choosing better food for yourself. Thank you for inspiring me to create these recipes for you! I wish you joyous health, today and always.

My hubs, Walker This book was possible because of my hungry, creative, sassy (yes, that's what we call him in the office) hubs, Walker. We created this book together—I developed the recipes (and many of them we'd been eating together for years) and cooked the food, he took the photos and then he ate the food. Well, I ate lots of food too, but if you could see the number of photos I took of Walker chowing down, you'd get a good laugh. I couldn't imagine a better life partner than my Walkman. Thank you for always challenging me and pushing me to be my best while making me laugh in the process. I love you to infinity and beyond!

Our daughter, Vienna You may have noticed I dedicated this cookbook to Vienna, and that's because many of these recipes were created with her in mind. She's my biggest inspiration. Having a child has been one of the best things to ever happen to me. Until I was pregnant with Vienna, it would never have occurred to me to consider putting a chicken fingers recipe in a cookbook. But everything changed when I realized that I needed to make food more accessible for people with little hands and smaller appetites than my husband and me. I'm grateful to have a human in my life who reminds me that life is full of so much possibility.

My mom (Susan) and my dad (Michael) I feel very fortunate that I've never had to persuade my parents to try a new superfood or recipe. They always welcome my ideas (which are sometimes very different than what they are used to) with open arms. My mom does most of the cooking for them, and she's always giving me ideas on how to make a recipe even better. She reviewed all these recipes and helped me when I started seeing double after staring at a computer screen too long. Thank you, Mom and Dad, for all your support today, tomorrow and always—I can count on you.

Carol Dano This book came to joyous life with Carol's creativity, eye for cool props and fabrics, and her genuine love for all things joyous. Working with her over the past decade has been nothing short of amazing, and I'm so grateful for her dedication, work ethic and hilariousness!

My right-hand lady, Rachel Molenda Our community manager at Joyous Health, Rachel held down the fort so I could be immersed in creating this book for five intense months. She's also one of the most pleasant, easygoing, adaptable people I know. We are so lucky to have her as part of the joyous team.

My other right-hand lady in the kitchen, Caroline Young Creating and cooking over 100 recipes for our book photoshoot was no small task. Thank you to Caroline for making it easier by being my right-hand lady in the kitchen, who never once complained even after standing for hour upon hour chopping, slicing, dicing, and sautéing, all the while with a smile.

Thank you to my publisher, Penguin Random House Canada, and to my editor, Andrea Magyar, for making this book a reality.

Thank you to all my recipe testers for your great ideas and for lending me your taste buds for five months. Laura, Erin, Andrea, Rachel, my mom—thank you!

INDEX